# Aroma~Care™

## How to Make Your Own Perfume

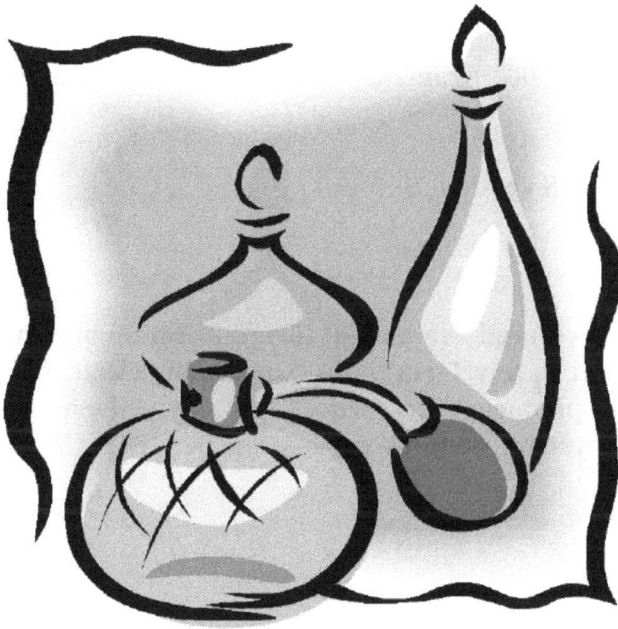

**Francine Milford**

Aroma~Care™ How to Make Your Own Perfume by Francine Milford

Aroma~Care™ is a series of instructional booklets on a variety of uses for essential oils.

FrancineMilford@cs.com
www.ReikiCenterofVenice.com
www.AromaCareBooks.com

ID: 978-0-6151-5171-7

Caution
The techniques, ideas, and suggestions presented in this book are not intended as a substitute for proper medical advice. Any application of the techniques, ideas, and suggestions in this book is at the reader's sole discretion and risk.

## Table of Contents

### Basic Concepts of Aromatherapy

### Scientific Principles

### Administration

## How to Make a Perfume

**Chapter One**
**History of Aromatherapy from Ancient to Modern Day Uses**


**What is Aromatherapy?**

The term "Aromatherapy" comes from two words, "Aroma" meaning scent and "Therapy" meaning a treatment for a physical or mental condition. Together, Aromatherapy means treating a physical or mental condition using scent. The scent of essential oils comes from plants that are valued for their therapeutic properties. These scents have been used for more than 5,000 years.

Aromatherapy comes from the premise that many illnesses were found to originate in the mind and that a holistic approach may be necessary for healing both body and mind. When essential oils are properly administered, they produce no harmful side effects and help to mobilize the body's own self-healing equilibrium or psychological well-being to regulate physical imbalances.

Essential oils can affect both the physical body and the spirit. Oils have the ability to directly affect the brain and many psychological and physiological processes. Use of aroma lamps, sprays, and inhalation devices bring the many properties of essential oils to the brain.

**Characteristics of Essential Oils**

Essential Oils are the *Essence* of the plant. Each plant has its own characteristics, personality, life force and energy (vibration). It is this essence that is the carrier of the plant's energy. This essence is the chemical make-up found in the plant itself. This make- up helps to protect the plant from invaders.

Essential Oils are more than 50 times more powerful in oil than herb form. Oils can be taken from various plant parts such as flowers, leaves, bark, seeds, berries, etc. It takes approximately 4,000 pounds of rose petals to create 1 pound of essential oil-that is one reason that some oils are priced more/less than other.

## How Essential Oils work

There are many ways that Essential oils can work on our body. One way is from it being absorbed through the skin. Through the

absorption process, essential oils are carrying to the tissues and organ systems of the body and are transported through the fluids of the body such in the lymph and blood systems. Another way essential oils work is through inhalation. When we inhale the aroma, we set into motion our olfactory system which begins with the aroma penetrating our mucus membrane and the hair-like structures of the olfactory nerves called cilia. Cilia relays this information to the brain which then responds to the stimuli by either becoming stimulated, relaxed, happy, sad, etc.

## Ancient Uses

6,000 B.C. - Egyptians were distilling their essential oils for use in perfumes and in burial rites, including (embalming the dead).

-Hippocrates, who has been called the 'Father of Medicine,' promoted daily bath and massages using oils.

-It was the Roman Physician, Discorides, that wrote down information for more than 500 medicinal plants.

5,000 B.C. - Chinese medicine was using plants for healing, beauty products, to make fragrant teas and rice (like jasmine), infused oils and incense and more.

1,000 B.C. - In Australia, the Aboriginal people used the Melaleuca species medicinally.

-Native American Indian Shamans in South America was using essential oils to perform their traditional healing work.

-North America, Native American Indians were burning herbs such as sage, cedar and sweetgrass to create a smoke that they used for purification is what is called smudging.

-Aztecs, Incas and Mayans used steam baths, massage and aromatherapy together. They created a Pinewood ointment that they rubbed on the chest for lung ailments, or elsewhere for muscle pain and aches.

- written work of herbalist Galen that set the standard for Europe for over 1,000 years.

-2,000 A.D. The King James Bible references more than 200 oils in the book.

## Modern Day Uses

-1700s. Distillation of plants and flowers was very popular and mostly used in Eau de Cologne and perfumes

-1709. Eau de Cologne-a blend of essential oils and 70/90% ethanol was created by Italian Perfumer.

-1187. Lab testing on antibacterial properties of essential oils.

-1920. Maurice Gattefosse-French perfume chemist-becomes known as the 'Father of Aromatherapy.' He records his research on the healing and antibacterial properties of oils in his book *'Gattefosse's Aromatherapie'*. The book was published in 1937 and is still in print today.

-1920s. French chemist Rene'-Maurice Gattefosse' published his findings in his new field of study that he called, 'L'*aromatherapie.*'

1950s. French biochemist, Marguerite Maury, used aromatherapy in the beauty industry.

-1958. Jean Valnet who started using essential oils in his practice and later he published the now classic book, *The Practice of Aromatherapy.*

-1992. King Tut's grave is opened and the world sees how long essential oil aromas last.

-present day. Tidewell Hospice & Pallative Care here in Florida realizes the importance of massage and essential oils and offer these services to their patients. They also offer classes to their staff in the use of aromatherapy. I even attended one of these classes myself as a massage therapist for which they gave me continuing education credits.

-present day. Many cleaning products contain essential oils such as pine, orange and lavender. Many hand, bath and body products contain essential oils.


## What to know before you purchase essential oils

Before you make your essential oil purchase, there are a few things that you should know and look out for. Below is a small list that I feel is important consumer information:

### Read the label.

Does the label read 'pure', 'genuine,' or 'fragrance'? If so, then you sure know the difference between them. 'Pure' can be a lot of different things to different companies. So don't base your purchase on this word alone. 'Fragrance' does NOT mean that you are purchasing essential oils.

If you are looking for essential oils, then be sure that the label reads, '100% essential oil' on it. Know where your supplier gets their essential oils and what extraction method that they use. Be aware of the companies ethical business standards, quality guarantees, customer support offerings, etc. We will cover more on this topic a little later in this course.

### Grade.

Essential oils sometimes come in what is called 'grades.' Lower grades of oils are sometimes sold as higher grades. We will cover this a little more in the next few pages.

### Extended.

I       f you read this on the label of essential oils then this means that the bottle contains a carrier oil (usually jojoba) to which some essential oil is added. I am finding this happening where generally the essential oil (such as rose) is so expensive that they add a few drops of it to jojoba in order to sell it the public at an affordable price.

### Testing.

The surest way to validate the quality of your essential oil is through a process called Gas Chromatography. This process reports on what chemical constituents are present and in what amounts and is used to verify whether a product reading, '100% pure essential oil' is really just that. We will cover this later on in this course.

### Folded.

This is the process of distilling oils several times in order to remove monoterpenes from the oil. This is usually performed on citrus oils.

### Rectified or Redistilled.

This is a process of removing a natural component from an essential oil. Some of these natural components include terpene and furocoumarin.

### Reconstituted.

This is where an essential oil has a natural or synthetic chemical component added to after they have been through the distillation process.

### Intuition and Instinct.

Trust your own instincts and sniff the essential oil. Does the essential oil feel that it has therapeutic value? Is it clear? Does the aroma linger? Our noses know what is real and what is not. Most people with allergies to chemical scents and perfumes, and I include myself in this group, will not have an allergic reaction to pure essential oils. The reason behind that is the fact that pure essential oils do not have the same protein structure as synthetic fragrances and our bodies know the difference between them. Our bodies will accent the protein structure of essential oils but not those of synthetic ones.

### Pricing.

One way to perhaps tell if an essential oil is 'real' or not is by its pricing.

Extremely Expensive oils: Rose, jasmine, melissa

Expensive: Frankincense, chamomile, sandalwood

Moderate: Lavender, peppermint, basil

Inexpensive: Eucalyptus, rosemary, orange

## Grades of Essential Oil

The first thing that I want to mention here is that there is NO such thing as a "therapeutic grade" essential oil. This is a coined phrase that has come from a pyramid-selling type of company that sells their essential oils. Some companies that are Multi-Level Marketing companies (MLMs) call their essential oils such names as "Therapeutic Grade" or "Pure Therapeutic Grade" or "Certified Pure Therapeutic Grade," etc. This is just their own private labeling brand and does not speak to a national or global standard.

Currently, there are no quality standards or governmental issues to authenticate or judge the quality or performance of essential oils. Hopefully that will change in the future, but for now, any company using these terms are just using them for advertising purposes and as a marketing ploy to lure potential customers in to buy their products. The only for you as the consumer to guarantee the quality of the essential oils that you are purchasing is by using Gas Chromatography and Mass Spectrometry (GC/MS). We will look at this topic a little later on in the course.

For your own information, I have listed below the 'grades' of essential oil that is being promoted by some of these companies. To be sure whether any one company is giving you what you are purchasing, you will have to contact that company directly and ask them questions. To date, there are essentially four grades of essential oils and they are designed by a letter, A through C, and Floral Water.

Grade A essential oils are pure therapeutic quality.
    Pure therapeutic quality
    Usually made from organically grown plants
    Distilled at proper temperatures using steam distillation
Grade B essential oils are food grade.
    Food grade
    May contain carrier oils, chemical additives, fertilizers, pesticides, synthetics, or synthetic extenders.
Grade C oils are perfume grade.
    Perfume grade
    Usually contain solvents

May contain the same type of adulterating chemicals as
listed in Grade B.
Floral Water is a byproduct of the distillation process.
By product of the distillation process


**Sources and origins of our Essential Oils**

Consumers of essential oils can receive their products from places all over the world. But how do these places affect the quality and constituents of the essential oil? What makes one source of essential oils better than another one?

To help answer these questions, Geoff Lyth from Quinessence Aromatherapy wrote an article titled, "Sources and Origins of our Essential Oils." For his own company, Lyth understands that it takes years of training and testing to learn about the various properties and the organic chemistry of a given species of plant.

Lyth sees that there are few companies that have been in business long enough to gain vital expertise in understanding the many genetic differences in the plant. There is much to learn about the many factors that affect the essential oil of a plant including where it was grown, how it was handled, how it was cultivated and so much more.

But knowing the origin of an essential oil will help you in selecting the right oils to use. An example of this is that if consumers know that the Lavender (Lavandula angustifolia) oil comes from France, then selecting a Lavender essential oil originating in another country may have different properties and as such had different results. This doesn't mean that Lavender coming from a different country is bad; it just means that it will potentially have a different chemistry, odor profile and even a different therapeutic action. Some basic essential oils and their country of origin include the following:

| Essential Oils | Latin Names | Origin |
| --- | --- | --- |
| Anise Star | Illicium verum | China |
| Basil* | Ocimum basilicum | Italy |
| Bay | Laurus nobilis | Morocco |
| Benzoin | Stryax benzoin | Sumatra |
| Bergamot | Citrus bergamia | Italy |
| Birch Sweet* | Betula Alba | USA |
| Black Pepper** | Piper nigrum | India |
| Cajeput | Melaleuca cajeputi | Indonesia |
| Cassia | Cinnamomum cassia | Vietnam |
| Carnation Absolute | Dianthus caryophyllus | Holland |
| Carrotseed | Daucus carota | France |
| Cedarwood* | Cedarus deodora | India |
| Chamomile German | Matricaria chamonilla | Hungary |
| Chamomile Roman* | Chameamelum nobile | Hungary |
| Cinnamon Leaf** | Cinnamomum verum | France |
| Citronella** | Cymbopogon nardus | Sri Lanka |
| Clary Sage* | Salvia sclarea | Bulgaria |
| Clove Bud** | Syzgium aromaticum | India |
| Coriander | Corriandrum sativum | Russia |
| Cypress* | Cupressus | France |
| Eucalyptus | Eucalyptus globulus | China |
| Fennel Sweet | Foeniculum v. dulce | France |
| Frankincense* | Boswellia carteri | Ethiopia |
| Geranium* | Peargoneum graveolens | Egypt |
| Ginger Root** | Zingiber officinalis | France |
| Grapefruit Pink | Citrus paradisi | France |
| Grapefruit White | Citrus racemosa | France |
| Hyssop* | Hyssopus officinalis | Europe |
| Jasmine Absolute* | Jasminum grandiflorum | France |
| Juniper Berry* | Juniperus communis | India |
| Lavender Bulgarian* | Lavandula angustifolia | Bulgaria |
| Lavender Croatian* | Lavandula officinalis | Croatia |

| | | |
|---|---|---|
| Lavender French* | Lavandula dentata | France |
| Lemon** | Citrus limonum | Italy |
| Lemon Eucalyptus** | Eucalyptus citriodora | Australia |
| Lemongrass** | Cymbopogon flexuous | India |
| Lime** | Citrus aurantifolia | Italy |
| Marjoram* | Thymus mastichina | Spain |
| Melissa Leaf | Melissa officinalis | Egypt |
| Mullein*/** | Verbascum thapsus | India |
| Myrrh* | Commiphora myrrha | Africa |
| Myrtle | Myrtus communis | France |
| Neroli | Citrus aurantium | France |
| Niaouli | Melaleuca viridiflora | New Caledonia |
| Nutmeg*/** | Myristica fragrans | Indonesia |
| Orange Sweet** | Citrus sinensis | Brazil |
| Origanum*/** | Origanum vulgare | France |
| Palmarosa | Cymbopogon martinii | India |
| Parsley | Petroselinum sativum | Egypt |
| Patchouli | Pogostemon cablin | Indonesia |
| Pennyroyal*/** | Mentha pulegium | France |
| Peppermint*/** | Menthe arvenisis | Japan |
| Petitgrain | Petitgrain bigarde | France |
| Pine (Long Leaf) | Pinus pinaster | USA |
| Pine (Scotch) | Pinus sylvestris | Hungary |
| Rose Damask Abs.* | Rosa damascena | Turkey |
| Rose Geranium* | Pelagonium graveolens | France |
| Rose Maroc Absolute* | Rosa centifolia | Morocco |
| Rosemary* | Rosmarinus officinalis | Spain |
| Rosewood | Aniba rosaeodora | Brazil |
| Sage*/** | Salvis officinalis | Croatia |
| Sandalwood Australian | Santalum spicatum | Australia |
| Sandalwood Mysore | Santalum album | East Indian |
| Tangerine | Citrus reticulata | Italy |
| Tea Tree | Melaleuca alternifolia | Australia |

| Thyme White* | Thymus vulgaris | France |
| Vanilla | Vanilla planifolia | Brazil |
| Vetiver | Vetiveria zizaniodes | Java |
| Violet Absolute | LeafViola odorata | France |
| Wintergreen*/** | Gaulgheria procumbens | India |
| Ylang Ylang | Cananga odorata | France |

* Avoid these Aromatherapy Essential Oils during pregnancy
**These Essential Oils can be skin irritants. Avoid if you have sensitive skin.

Aromatherapy Essential Oils are best kept in amber glass bottles to protect them from direct light and heat.
www.AromaCareBooks.com

**Chapter Two**
**Client Assessment**

The word 'assessment' refers to the process of appraising a client's condition based on both their subjective reporting and your objective findings. This is accomplished in the consultation.

Before and Aromatherapist begins working with a new client, time is set aside for the aromatherapy consultation. This consultation provides the therapists with unique insights into the current needs of the new client. Consultations can be done either in person or on the telephone. When a client comes in person, the client's demeanor can give the Aromatherapist additional information about the health and wellbeing of their client. The Aromatherapist can take a look at the client's skin color and pallor, the client's eyes, the feel of the skin, the way the client walks (fast, slow, limping, crooked, etc.).

A typical consultation will last between 15 minutes to 60 minutes. This session will set up the client-practitioner relationship needed to establish goals and treatment strategies. The Aromatherapist will use this time to identify any underlying issues and prioritize the needs of the systems of the body. The therapist will also look at building a treatment plan and determine the goals for the client, and how long it should take for the client to see any improvement.

The consultation generally begins with the client filling out a detailed client In-take (like the one that follows at the end of this chapter). The In-take should include the following information:
Client Basic Information (name, age, sex, marital status, occupation, address, telephone number, allergies, medications, health history, current health, etc.)
Reason client is seeking aromatherapy
Client's preference for aromatherapy application
Any contraindications

**There are three major components to the in-person consultation. These components are:**
**Observation**
**Interviewing**
**Evaluation**

## Observation

By studying and monitoring your client, Aromatherapists will take into account several factors of their client before deciding on an Aromatherapy blend. Some of the things that the therapists will notice will be the emotional state of their client. Is their client jumpy and easily agitated or are they subdued and lethargic? Are they overweight or underweight? Do they look like they are retaining fluids or have edema? Take a look at their posture. Are they standing straight and tall and move from their hips when they walk, or are they slumped over or look off balance?

Take a look at their muscle tone. Are the muscles taut and is the skin healthy looking or do their muscles sag and their skin look yellowish or pale? Look at your clients' eyes. Do the whites of the eyes look white and clear and do their pupils look moist and shiny or do are the whites of the eyes actually yellowed or bloodshot and are their pupils dry or uneven looking?

Notice your client's voice as they speak. Do they speak with confidence and positivity or is their speech uneven, unsure or even slurred? How is your client communicating their needs and situation to you? Are they hesitating to give up any information or are they like a never ending waterfall of data?

For a successful consultation, it is important for you, the therapists, to take plenty of notes on what you are observing about your client's behavior as listed above. Take note of their expressions and body language.

Do they appear open to sharing their information with you or do they sit back, inattentive and uninvolved in their own treatment plan. Be sure that you implore using active listening techniques which means that not only will you ask open and closed questions, but that you will listen fully to the answers that are given to you.

When you do receive answers from your client, be sure to paraphrase the answers back to you client for verification and or additional information. Be sure to maintain eye contact with your client as it shows that you are involved and care about what they have to say to you.

Also be aware of your non-verbal communication with your client. If you glance at your watch or on the clock on the wall, then you are signaling to your client that you are inpatient. If you glance at your phone that just 'buzzed' a message because you were not professional enough to turn it off, you may give your client the impression that you are not totally in tune with them and their situation, or that you would rather be somewhere else and doing something else. Tapping your pen or nails on the table would also send the message that you are bored with the conversation or impatient with the client.

Be sure that you give your client some feedback to any questions that they are asking you. If you don't know the answer to a particular question, then be honest with them and tell them that. Also be sure to tell them that you will find the information for them and will send it to them, call them with it, or have it ready for them on their next visit. Never judge your client's history or situation as being bad, or good. Try to remain impartial to the issues at hand.

You must also take your client's age and experiences in hand when deciding on what essential oils to blend for them. Always dress and act professionally, maintain eye contact, use proper body language, respect your boundaries and your client's boundaries (which we discuss later in the manual), provide feedback, watch your non-verbal communication, and be observant. One great way to see how you are performed is to go through a mock interview with a friend and video tape the session. When you watch back the session, you will learn a lot about your own strengths and weaknesses.

**Interviewing**

Therapists will look over the information that client has filled out on the Client In-take form, along with information form observing the client. If the therapist fills that there are areas of information that are incomplete, or that a particular statement needs to be clarified, then the therapist will ask the client open or closed questions.

Closed questions are questions that be easily answered with a 'yes' or 'no' answer or a single word or phrase. Ask closed questions when you want a specific, quick, easy fact and you want to maintain control of the conversation. Open questions are questions that can receive a long answer. Ask open questions when you want your client to think or reflect upon something, give you their feelings or opinions, or when you want them to elaborate.

Open questions usually begin with words such as 'What if' and 'How would you' or 'Why did you' or even 'Tell me how' or 'Describe to me.' The additional information that you gather from the interviewing process will help you in determining how to best help your client. Additional questions may be in regards to any known allergic reactions to plants, nuts, ragweed, flowers, grains, herbs, trees, spices, etc.

At this time, it is also important for me to find out what my client expectations are from me and Aromatherapy in general. What have they tried on their own and what have been their experiences in the past with other therapists and therapies? Does the client has realistic expectations of both my abilities and scope of practice, as well as, what essential oils can and cannot do? If I feel that the client is being unrealistic in the expectations, then this is a time that I use in educating the client in what I, and essential oils, can do for them. If the client agrees with these new realistic expectations, then I will continue with the session. If the client does not agree with these realistic expectations, then I will either close the session or ask some open questions such as, "Why do you believe that this essential oil will perform as you believe?" or "Where have you read the information or data that you believe? This usually helps you in determining the ultimate success you
will have.


**Evaluation**

Following the consultation, the Aromatherapist will make an assessment of the client's need be going over the information from the client in-take form and observations, and from asking additional questions, etc. The Aromatherapist will then create a blend for the client that will address the client's specific needs.

When finished, the therapist will set out a treatment planning and recommendation for the client. Expectations will be established and how treatment evaluation and review will be taken (weekly, monthly, etc.). Follow-up sessions will be discussed and planned out. Aftercare advice will also be given on follow-up sessions.

The therapist will customize an individual blend for the client, as well as, how the client is to administer the blend (massage, bath, compresses, etc.) The Therapist should give the client a hand out on how often the client is to use the blend and what to do in case of accidental eye contact or ingestion. I like to include contact numbers on this sheet of paper for my own contact information, as well as, poison centers and hospitals.

It is important for the therapist to be contacted if the blend is not working as planned or if something has happened that has made a significant change to the situation, such as being hospitalized or given new medications from your primary healthcare provider, as this may affect you using a given Aromatherapy blend. It is also important to know if the client presents with an allergic reaction to the blend that you have made for them.

A good therapist will document the measurements of the ingredients that they use in a blend for their client. In this way, if they have to replicate the blend again for their client, they will be able to. Be sure to add this document to the client's records along with future notes that speak to the effectiveness of the blend and treatment. You never know if you will use this information in the future for a research project, so be sure that all of your documentation is complete and current.

## Client In-take Form

Date_____

Name_____

Address _____

City _____ State _____ Zip Code _____

Telephone(___) _____

Email Address _____

Birthdate _____ Sex _____

Reason for Visit _____

List all of your Medications:_____

How often do you move your bowels every day? _____

How much water do you drink in one day? _____

How much sugar do you consume in one day? _____

How much meat do you consume in one week? _____

How much white flour do you consume? _____

How many dairy products do you eat? _____

Do you feel stressed? Explain_____

Do you have trouble sleeping? _____


Are you pregnant or nursing? _____

Do you have any emotional concerns or needs?_____

Do you have any oils that you like? _____

Do you have any oils that you don't like? _____

The BODY SYSTEM'S QUESTIONNAIRE is below

Client: Circle all numbers in the row that relates to your current issue.

| Body Systems | 1 | 2 | 3 | 4 | 5 | 6 | 7 | 8 | 9 | 10 | 11 |
|---|---|---|---|---|---|---|---|---|---|---|---|
| Abdominal Pain or Discomfort | x | x | x | | | | | | | | |
| Acid indigestion or heartburn | x | | | | | | | | | | |
| Anxiety, nervousness or tension | x | | | | | | x | x | | | |
| Allergies, Asthma, Hay fever | x | x | | X | | | | | | | |
| Anemia | x | | | | | x | | | | x | |
| Bad breath (Halitosis) or body odor | | | x | | X | | | | | | |
| Burning or painful urination | | | | | X | | | | | | |
| Cold hands and feet | | | | | | x | | x | | | |

| | | | | | | | | | | | |
|---|---|---|---|---|---|---|---|---|---|---|---|
| Colitis or other bowel irritations | | x | x | | | | | | | X | |
| Constipation or dry stools | | | x | | | | x | | | | |
| Dark circles or puffiness under eyes | | x | | | x | | | x | | | |
| Dizziness or light headedness | | | | | | x | | x | | | |
| Excess mucous production | | | x | x | | | | x | | | |
| Fatigue or low energy levels | | x | x | | | x | x | x | | x | |
| Frequent backache | | | | | x | | | x | x | | |
| Frequent cough | | | | x | | | | x | | x | |
| Frequent infections | | | | x | | | | x | | x | |
| Frequent urinary tract infections | | | | | x | | | x | | | |
| General weakness or chronic illness | x | | | | | | | x | | x | x |
| Heart Problems | | | | | | x | | x | | | |
| High blood pressure | | | | | x | x | x | x | | | |
| High cholesterol | | | x | | | x | | x | | | |
| Infertility | | | | | | | | | | | x |
| Insomnia | | | x | | | | x | x | | | |
| Intestinal gas, bloating, flatulence | x | x | x | | | | | | | | |
| Joint pain, arthritis or gout | | | | | x | | | | x | | |
| Leg cramps or pains | | | | | x | | | | x | | |
| Migraine Headaches | | | x | | | x | x | | | | x |
| Muscle aches and pains, stiffness | | x | x | | x | | | | x | x | |
| PMS | | | | | | | x | | | | x |
| Sinus Congestion | | | x | x | | | | | | x | |
| Skin problems | | | x | | x | | | | x | x | x |
| Stress | | | | | | | x | x | | | x |
| Swollen lymph glands (immune system) | | x | | x | | | | | | x | |
| Varicose Veins | | x | | | x | | | | x | | |
| Grand Totals | | | | | | | | | | | |

| | Digestive | Hepatic | Intestinal | Respiratory | Urinary | Circulation | Glandular Structural | Immune | Reproductive |
|---|---|---|---|---|---|---|---|---|---|
| | | | | | | | | | |

For the Professional to fill out
1-Add the total of the circled numbers in each column in the Grand Total above.
2-List the Body Systems from the previous chart that your client circled from 1-10.

(1 will represent the column with the MOST circled x's in it and 10 is the least)
Write down the body system in order from the most x's to the least.
1.
2.
3.
4.
5.
6.
7.
8.
9.
10.
11.


**NOTE**: Now you have a very good ideal of which of your client's body systems are in most need of help. You have the choice of working on one system at a time, or creating a blend for your client that will take care of several body systems at one time. As each situation and client is unique, you will have to make your best educated guess on how you would like to proceed with your client. If you need help on a particular client, you can drop me an email at FrancineMilford@cs.com.

The Blend Ingredients:
Essential Oils and Number of drops used

_____

_____

_____

_____

_____

Carrier Used _____

Method of Application _____

Length of time to use blend _____

Precautions and Contraindications _____

Additional Recommendations and Information:

_____

_____

Follow-up Date _____


Additional Notes:

**Medical History**

It is important for you, the therapist, to discover any and all prescription drugs, over the counter medication, and supplements that you client is taking. You will need to know these things so that you do not offer your client an essential oil that can harm them. Below is a list of some popular medications and supplements and their potential negative interactions with essential oils.

Essential oils are fat soluble and can be accessed by the cells in the human body and metabolized by the body. So when there are other drugs present in the body, the active agents of the essential oil may react with that drug in either a positive, negative or neutral way.

**Drug Interactions-(Prescription/ Nonprescription)**

I encounter the same problems with using essential oils as I do with using herbs in the healing process. Those problems surround people who believe that because essential oils and herbs come from plants and as such are considered 'natural' products, that they can't harm you. This is simply not true. I always treat herbs and essential oils as medicine. In doing so, it helps to remind you to handle and dose with care. You can cause harm if you do not take proper care in preparing blends for your clients.

Some drug interactions may occur during the simple application of just inhaling an essential oil. A highly volatile oil such as Peppermint oil can cause increased lung permeability of nicotine and slow the ability to clear nicotine from the body (Harris, 2008).

Exercise caution when using essential oils in topical application around drug injection side, open cuts or wounds, and around patches (estrogen or nicotine). The wintergreen essential oil has a cortisone-like action because it has a high methyl salicylate, so I would avoid giving wintergreen to clients who are already taking cortisone either internally or topically. In Europe, it is common to see essential oils being given orally, vaginally or rectally. In the United States, we have chosen not to use essential oils orally as this usage must be closely monitored by a medical practitioner or a professional Aromatherapist.

| Essential Oil | Avoid Mixing with | Main Body System |
|---|---|---|
| Rosemary | Anesthesia, barbituates, May inactivate antibiotics Sedatives (such as barbiturates, benzodiazepines, anesthetics) | Respiratory, Immune |
| Eucalyptus | Anesthesia, barbituates Sedatives (such as barbiturates, benzodiazepines, anesthetics) | Respiratory |
| Ravinstara | Anesthesia, barbituates Sedatives (such as barbiturates, benzodiazepines, anesthetics) May inhibit platelet aggregation, May exacerbate blood-thinning action of drugs | Respiratory |
| Bay laurel | Anesthesia, barbituates Sedatives (such as barbiturates, benzodiazepines, anesthetics) | Respiratory |
| Wintergreen | Anticoagulant drugs, asthmatics, aspirin allergies. Not for people with ADD/ADHD May cause hemorrhaging in users taking Warfarin (Coumadin, aspirin or Heparin) | Respiratory, Immune, Cardiovascular |
| Birch | Anticoagulant drugs, asthmatics, aspirin allergies. Not for people with ADD/ADHD May cause hemorrhaging in users taking Warfarin (Coumadin, aspirin or Heparin) | Respiratory, Immune, Cardiovascular |
| Clove, Clove Bud | Anticoagulant drugs, asthmatics, aspirin allergies (Warfarin, Coumadin, aspirin or Heparin) Antidepressants (MAOI or SSRI drugs, Quinidine, Floxetine and Paroxetine, Codeine and | Respiratory, Immune, Cardiovascular |

| | Tamoxifen)<br>possible cardiovascular changes<br>prostaglandin inhibitors | |
|---|---|---|
| Thyme | Avoid if you have bleeding disorders, major surgery, childbirth, peptic ulcer or hemophilia<br>(Warfarin, Coumadin, aspirin or Heparin)<br>prostaglandin inhibitors<br>May inhibit platelet aggregation, May exacerbate blood-thinning action of drugs | Respiratory, Immune, Cardiovascular |
| Oregano | (Warfarin, Coumadin, aspirin or Heparin)<br>Avoid if you have bleeding disorders, major surgery, childbirth, peptic ulcer or hemophilia<br>May inhibit platelet aggregation, May exacerbate blood-thinning action of drugs | Respiratory, Immune, Cardiovascular |
| Cinnamon Leaf | Anticoagulant drugs, asthmatics, aspirin allergies<br>May inhibit platelet aggregation, May exacerbate blood-thinning action of drugs | Respiratory, Immune, Cardiovascular |
| Allspice Berry | Anticoagulant drugs, asthmatics, aspirin allergies | Respiratory, Immune, Cardiovascular |
| Pimento Berry | Anticoagulant drugs, asthmatics, aspirin allergies | Respiratory, Immune, Cardiovascular |
| Niaouli | Increases penicillin and streptomycin | Immune |
| Lemon | May inactivate antibiotics | Immune |
| Lemongrass | May inactivate antibiotics<br>Antidepressants such as Bupropion which inhibits CYP2B6 enzyme | Immune |

| | may influence blood sugar levels | |
|---|---|---|
| Lemon Balm | May inactivate antibiotics | Immune |
| Citrus Eucalyptus Eucalyptus | May inactivate antibiotics Sedatives (such as barbiturates, benzodiazepines, anesthetics) | Immune |
| Citronellal | May inactivate antibiotics | Immune |
| Cinnamon Bark | May inactivate antibiotics may influence blood sugar levels May inhibit platelet aggregation, May exacerbate blood-thinning action of drugs | Immune |
| Orange | May inactivate antibiotics | Immune |
| Ginger | May inactivate antibiotics | Immune |
| Melissa | May inactivate antibiotics | Immune |
| Peppermint | May inactivate antibiotics, Avoid smoking/nicotine calcium channel blocker (felodipine) | Immune, Respiratory, Digestive, cardiovascular |
| Sage | May inactivate antibiotics | Immune |
| Spike Lavender | May inactivate antibiotics | Immune |
| Pennyroyal | May exacerbate glutathione depletion (Acetaminophen) | |
| Nutmeg | Antidepressants (MAOI or SSRI drugs, Quinidine, Floxetine and Paroxetine, Codeine and Tamoxifen) possible cardiovascular changes | |
| Holy Basil | Antidepressants (MAOI or SSRI drugs, Quinidine, Floxetine and Paroxetine, Codeine and Tamoxifen) | |
| Bay (West Indian) | Antidepressants (MAOI or SSRI drugs, Quinidine, Floxetine and Paroxetine, Codeine and Tamoxifen) prostaglandin inhibitors | |
| Parsley | Antidepressants (MAOI or SSRI | |

| | | |
|---|---|---|
| Seed | drugs, Quinidine, Floxetine and Paroxetine, Codeine and Tamoxifen) | |
| German Chamomile | Inhibit metabolizing enzymes (CYP2D6) <br> may potentiate the actions of some antidepressants | |
| Blue Tansy | Inhibit metabolizing enzymes (CYP2D6) <br> may potentiate the actions of some antidepressants | |
| Yarrow | Inhibit metabolizing enzymes (CYP2D6) <br> may potentiate the actions of some antidepressants | |
| Balsam Poplar | Inhibit metabolizing enzymes (CYP2D6) <br> may potentiate the actions of some antidepressants | |
| Geranium | may influence blood sugar levels | |
| Tumeric | may influence blood sugar levels | |
| Melissa | may influence blood sugar levels | |
| Lemon Myrtle | may influence blood sugar levels <br> May inhibit platelet aggregation, May exacerbate blood-thinning action of drugs | |
| Anise, Star Anise | may influence blood sugar levels <br> Anti-diuretic properties <br> May inhibit platelet aggregation, May exacerbate blood-thinning action of drugs | |
| Cassia | May influence blood sugar levels <br> May inhibit platelet aggregation, May exacerbate blood-thinning action of drugs | |
| Fennel | May inhibit platelet aggregation, May exacerbate blood-thinning action of drugs | |
| Lavandin | May inhibit platelet aggregation, | |

|  | May exacerbate blood-thinning action of drugs |  |
|---|---|---|
| Marigold | May inhibit platelet aggregation, May exacerbate blood-thinning action of drugs |  |
| Patchouli | May inhibit platelet aggregation, May exacerbate blood-thinning action of drugs |  |
| Tarragon | May inhibit platelet aggregation, May exacerbate blood-thinning action of drugs |  |
| Sedative Oils | May cause too much sleepiness CNS depressants clonazepam (Klonopin), lorazepam (Ativan), phenobarbital (Donnatal), zolpidem (Ambien) |  |

**The Initial Consultation**

The first thing that you should do before you begin the initial consultation is to escort your new client to a room that is quiet and private. This is a sensitive matter and should be kept private. Be sure that there is adequate lighting for reading and writing. Be sure that the client feels safe and comfortable. Offer a glass of water if you like. Be sure that you will not be distracted during this time with knocks on the door or with phone calls. This can be very disruptive to the consultation and may send a signal to your new client that you are just not that interested in giving them any personal time.

During the initial consultation, you will have your new client fill out proper documentation in the form of the Client In-take form. You will then write down any of your observations about your client such as their postural analysis, muscle tone, weight, edema, skin sensitivities, allergies, the tone of their voice, their current lifestyle, age, overall health, medication contraindications, and your client's expectations.

The next part of the consultation is finding out what problem they want to deal with first. Which problem made them come to see you in the first place? You will them decide on creating a blend to address your client's specific needs and in what form the application of the blend will take (bath, massage, etc.). Be sure that everything is in writing and that you get your client to sign the form. Date the form. While a client may have many issues when they come to see you, I prefer to work on one issue at a time, if possible. It isn't always possible as several issues can tied in together. But I often let the client choose which issue is the one that they would like most to work on first.

The last part of the consultation session will be me going over the client's expectations for the treatment session to see if it is realistic. If it is not, then I will use this as an opportunity to educate the client on what is, and is not, realistic goal setting.

If a client refuses to fill out the client in-take form, then I will not work with them and I will send them home. I am a professional and as such, I must act accordingly. How can they respect me if I don't even respect my own profession? If they are serious about seeking professional help for their situation, then they will fill out the form. This speaks to my own liability of having a signed consent form from my clients too as we will discuss later on in this manual. We will now take a look at the informed consent form and why this is something important to have signed.

**Informed Consent**

The informed consent is a client's authorization for professional services based on the information given to them by the therapist. This must be signed by the client after it has been filled out by the therapist. This form will include the therapist's credentials, education and school attended.

Also listed will be any diplomas or certificates or licenses that the therapist has. This will serve as an opportunity for the therapist to lay a foundation of professionalism with the client and to display the therapist's ability to perform the required treatment plan.

Also listed on the informed consent form will be a description of the modalities that will be used, along with the expectations and potential benefits of using said modalities.

In this way, the client will better understand what a potential outcome and result from treatment and what is not.

The form will also contain potential risks and negative side effects of the modalities to be used. In this way, the client will be better able to make a wise and informed decision about their own health care needs. A statement of scope of practice will assure the client that the client does not diagnose a medical condition or prescribe services for medical treatments.

There will also be a *right of refusal* clause in the form where the client has the right to terminate the session for any reason and refuse to be treated by the therapist. This can be done either verbally or written. This works both ways to as you can stop working with a client who make you feel uncomfortable or makes sexual advances towards you. Part of this clause may include information for the client to use in reporting you to the professional board responsible for governing your actions as a therapist.

There should be information on how the client's information and records will be used and stored by you and your facility. You can view HIPAA guidelines to help you create the correct working.

Lastly, there should a paragraph on your office policies and procedures as they deal with client-therapist boundaries, dual relationships, fee schedules and payments, returned checks, canceled payments and missed appointments.

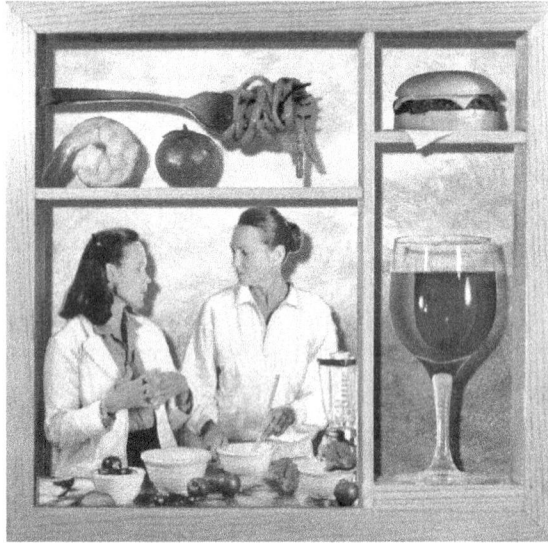

## How to Conduct the Consultation

Have the client fill out a client intake form. If you do not have one, one has been enclosed for you to use with this course.

After the client has filled out the form, look it over and verify the information (to be sure that the client has not made a mistake in filling out the information).

If you have any questions about the information that you are reading, now is the time to verify it with the client.

Ask any additional questions that you feel will help you to set up a plan of action for your client.

Be sure to ask the client what aromas that he/she likes and dislikes.

Begin with the focus of the blend-what goals or actions do you want to help the client achieve first. Having a focus to the blend will help you to narrow down your choices of essential oils that you will use. (A worksheet is included in this manual).

Then write down all of the essential oils that help you to accomplish your goal.

Now that you have your list of essential oils, cross off those that may have contraindications for your client-you can use your reference books to help you here.

Continue to cross essential oils off your list until you have narrowed down your selection to five or seven.

With the five or seven oils that you have, ask the client to sniff each to see which ones the client like, and which one they don't. At the end, be sure to have no more than 5 essential oils left.

Now, decide on which application you will use. With you have the client massage the oils into their bodies? Use compresses? Use a room mist?

After you have decided what application you will use with you client, you can now decide on which carrier oil you will use. Be sure to omit any and all carriers that may be contraindicated for your client. (Like peanut oil for people with nut allergies).

After deciding upon the use and carrier, you will need to decide how many drops of each essential oil you will need to create your blend. A chart is available on the following pages. Be sure to write down how many drops of each essential oil your will use into your notebook so that you can recreate the blend again in the future if you need to.

Blends essential oils first and then add your selected carrier. Shake gently to blend.

Sniff your blend to be sure that you are happy with the result. If you are, then have your client sniff the blend to see their reactions. Don't be surprised if you will have to add an additional drop of oil here or there to please the client's sense of smell.

With your blend completed, create a label with the following information on it:

- Name of the Blend
- Date of the Blend
- Essential oils included in the blend
- ype of carrier
- Directions for use
- How long to use
- Warnings such as 'Keep out of the reach of Children,' etc.
- Protocol to follow in case client accidently gets oil in their eye

Be sure to call your client in a few days to see how the product is working or you can set up a follow up date with your client before they leave you (say in one week). This will give you time to see if your blend is doing the job you were hoping for. If it is not, then you can revisit the situation on the next client visit.

Keep good notes on your client's reaction to the blends that you create. Make it a habit to track your results as this may lead to valuable research findings in the future.

## Contraindications

**Safety Guidelines and Contraindications of Essential Oils**

Because essential oils are popping up on shelves everywhere, the public needs to learn more about how and when to use these oils in a safe environment. Through a lack of knowledge, many people are being hurt by using essential oils. So please, educate yourself on the proper use of essential oils before using them on yourself and others.

**General Do's and Don't's**

- Do not take essential oils internally
- Keep essential oils out of the reach of children and pets
- Keep essential oils out of your eyes and mucous membranes
- Always dilute essential oils in a carrier oil (never apply oils directly to your skin)
- Be sure to use 100% pure essential oils.
- If you are taking Staten medications-avoid hepatoxic oils such as grapefruit.
- Remember that citrus oils are photosensitive. Stay out of sunlight for 12 hours after applying essential oils. Also, avoid tanning beds when using citrus oils.
- Asthma sufferers should avoid steam inhalation as this may irritate and aggravate the mucus membranes. Avoid essential oil of thyme.
- Avoid prolonged use of essential oils. Have 5-6 days on and take 1-2 days off.
- Avoid the essential oil of pine if you have prostate concerns.
- Store essential oils in colored glass containers out of direct sunlight.
- Be sure to use proper dosages for children and pets-do not use adult dosages.
- Use proper ventilation when using essential oils over a long period of time.

- Be sure to perform a Patch Test on yourself before applying essential oils to your entire body, especially if you have sensitive skin.
- Always check with your client about their past reactions to using essential oils.
- Refrigerate carrier oils to prevent them from becoming rancid.
- Old oils are more prone to cause skin reactions. Throw these oils out. Some oils like patchouli and sandalwood get better with age-most do not.
- If you keep a bird in your home, stay away from using essential oils in a diffuser.
- Use caution during pregnancy and while nursing. Safe essential oils include lavender, mandarin and Roman Chamomile.
- If you are allergic to foods like oranges, etc., then you will be potentially allergic to the oils of these products.
- While some oils are effective is used sparingly, they become less effective is you use them too often without a rest.

Consider any cold pressed citrus oil a potential photosensitizer. Steam distilled citrus oils, on the other hand, do not carry this risk. St. John's Wort CO2 and infused oil are also photosensitizers.

Some oils are so dangerous that we have asked you to stay away from using such as: Benzoin, Birch, Bitter Almond, Calamus, Yellow Camphor, Mugwort, Mustard, Rue, Sassafras, Southernwood, Tansy, Thuja, Wintergreen, Horseradish, Wormwood, Verbena, Bay Laurel, Mimosa, Lovage, Tolu Balsam, Ragetes, Peru Balsam, Galbanum Resin, Hyacinth, Oakmoss Concrete, Fig Leaf Absolute.

| Essential Oil | Avoid |
| --- | --- |
| Basil | Avoid during pregnancy, epilepsy, sensitive skin |
| Bergamot | Photosensitivity |
| Cassia | Avoid direct sunlight, photosensitivity |
| Citrus | Avoid direct sunlight |
| Clary Sage | Avoid during pregnancy (until labor), don't drink alcohol, estrogenic cancers |

| | |
|---|---|
| Clove | Avoid during pregnancy, skin sensitivity |
| Coriander | Avoid during pregnancy, avoid using too much at one time, kidney problems |
| Fennel | Avoid during pregnancy, people with seizures |
| Geranium | Low blood pressure, estrogenic cancers |
| Ginger | Sensitive skin |
| Hyssop | Avoid during pregnancy, seizures |
| Jasmine | Avoid during pregnancy, |
| Juniper | Kidney problems |
| Lemon | Photosensitivity |
| Lemongrass | Avoid during pregnancy, Sensitive skin |
| Lime | Photosensitivity |
| Marjoram | Drowsiness, diminish sex drive, decrease sexual function, numb erotic sensations |
| Melissa | Sensitive skin |
| Myrtle (lemon) | Avoid during pregnancy, |
| Myrrh | Avoid during pregnancy, |
| Oregano | Avoid during pregnancy, skin irritation |
| Patchouli | Photosensitivity |
| Peppermint | Avoid during pregnancy, Dilute for high blood pressure |
| Pine | High blood pressure |
| Roman Chamomile | Avoid during pregnancy (until labor), drowsiness |
| Rosemary | Avoid during pregnancy, high blood pressure, epilepsy |
| Rose | Estrogenic cancers |
| Sage | Avoid during pregnancy, seizures, high blood pressure |
| Sandalwood | Kidney problems |
| Sassafras | Carcinogenic |
| Tea Tree | Avoid during pregnancy, high blood pressure |
| Thyme | Avoid during pregnancy, sensitive skin, high blood pressure |
| Orange (wild) | Avoid direct sunlight |
| Ylang ylang | Low blood pressure |

**NOTES:**

**Chapter Three**
**Botany**


Botany, also called plant biology, is the science of plant life. A botanist is a scientist who studies plant biology. Botanists study some 400,000 species of living organism. Botany actually has its beginning from people who use to identity and cultivate plants for healing call herbalist. Their efforts to identify plants that were medicinal, edible and poisonous were catalogued into collections which were the beginnings of plant taxonomy. On such collections was created by Carl Linnaeus in 1753 and is still in use today.

Modern botany uses new techniques to study plants and analyzes plant chemistry using microscopy and live cell imagine. Botany today looks at the plant chemistry, chromosome number, enzymes, proteins, DNA sequences, etc., to better classify plants.

Botany is concerned with the range and diversity of organisms and their relationships in order to determine evolutionary history. Biological classification is the method by which botanists group organisms into categories such as genera or species and is a form of scientific taxonomy. Carolus Linnaeus grouped species according to shared physical characteristics. This became the beginning of modern taxonomy which now uses DNA sequences as data. The classification order is as follows:

Kingdom
Phylum (or Division )
Class
Order
Family
Genus (plural genera)-First word is capitalized and second is
        lowercase and all is italicized.
Species


To avoid confusion over using a variety of essential oils taken from similar plants, the industry uses Latin names for plant classification. The science of plant classification is called *Taxonony*.

Taxonomy is important because not only will it help you to distinguish one essential oil from another, but also what plant properties you will be getting as each species may offer different therapeutic values.

It is important for you to know not just the common name of the essential oil that you are using, but also its botanical name. In that way, you can be sure that you are using the correct plant and part of the plant to accomplish the result and outcomes that you want to.

Latin names of plants are written as follows:
Families
Genus-(first part of name and first word is capitalized)
Species
Subspecies
Cultivars and varieties
Chemotypes

**Families**

In biology, the word 'family' represents a taxonomic group that contains one or more genera. Did you know that there are at least three botanical families to the 'chamomile' plant? We have roman, german and moroccan. Each of these plants has different properties and constituents even though they belong to the same botanical family.

To discover more on specific plants, there are several databases that you can go to and look up information on specific plants. One such database is from the University of Florida and can be accessed at: http://edis.ifas.ufl.edu/topic_plant_families.

This database went online in 1995 first as the Florida Agricultural Information Retrieval System (FAIRS) and then three years later changed its name to the Extension Data Information Source (EDIS). It is now considered the single source for all Extension publications and a comprehensive, single-source repository for all peer reviewed publications for free distribution on the web. Funding is provided through the University of Florida Institute of Food and Agricultural Science.

Another free website is from the USDA, Natural Resources Conservation Service at http://www.plants.usda.gov/classification.html. Here you can look up specific information on any number of plants.

In botany, these are the plant families associated with essential oils:

Ericaceae-the 'heather' family.
Betulaceae-the 'birch' family.
Valerianaceae- Now part of the <u>Caprifoliaceae</u> family. 'honeysuckle' family.
Verbenaceae-the 'verbena' family.
Cistaceae-the 'rock rose' family.
Cruciferae-the 'cabbage' gamily.
Liliaceae-the 'lily' family.
Iridaceae-the 'iris' family.
Araceae-the 'inflorescence' family.
Palmae-the 'palm tree' family.
Cyperaceae-'sedges' family.
Moraceae-the 'mulberry' or 'fig' family.
Aristolochiaceae-the 'birthwort' family.
Chenopodiaceae-the 'goosefoot' family.
Ranunculaceae-the 'crowfoot' family.
Euphorbiaceae-the 'spurge' family.
Malvaceae-the 'mallows' family.
Ulmaceae-the 'elm' family.
Podocarpaceae-the 'evergreen' family.
Pinaceae-the 'pine' family.
Taxodiaceae-the 'coniferous' family.
Cupressacaea-the 'cypress' family.

## Genus

In biology, the word 'genus' is a taxonomic rank used in classifying living organisms. It is placed below family and above species on the hierarchical scale. The composition of a genus is determined by a taxonomist. The scientific name of a genus is always capitalized. This name may also be called the 'generic name' or 'generic epithet.'

**Species**

An example of an essential oil with different species is one of my personal favorite-Eucalyptus essential oil. Some of the names that you may encounter would be the standard, *Eucalyptus globulus,* or it could be *Eucalyptus citriodora* and *Eucalyptus*

Another consideration to keep in mind is that different species also come with different safety guidelines and uses. An example of one such essential oil is Basil. Sweet Basil, *Ocimum basilicum* var. *album* contains less phenolic ethers than its counterpart, Exotic Basil, *Ocimum basilicum* var. *basilicum.*

**Cultivars and Varieties**

A cultivar is a plant that was selected because of its desirable characteristics (such as resistance to disease, aroma, color, etc.) and maintained by propagation. Examples of this include food crops planted for agricultural, garden plants like roses, camellias and rhododendrons and trees used in forestry that were selected for enhanced quality and yield of timber.

A cultivar name consists of a botanical name (genus, species, infraspecific taxon) followed by a cultivar epithet that is enclosed by single quotes with each of the words within the epithet capitalized. An example of a cultivar name is as follow:

*Cryptomeria japonica* 'Elegans'

In botany, the word 'variety' is a taxonomic rank below that of a species. It can have an appearance that is distinct from other varieties and it is usually grown geographically separate from other species. Varieties are represented in a three-part infraspecific name. An example would be: The variety *Escobaria vivipara* var. *arizonica* is from Arizona and the *Escobaria vivipara* var. *neo-mexicana* is from New Mexico, but when they meet, they integrate.

**Plant Origin and Chemotypes**

Where the essential oil comes from can also affect the quality and therapeutic value of the oil. A good example for this is the Sandalwood tree which grows in India but also is being grown now in Australia and other areas of the world. But different minerals exist in the soils of different areas so this will affect the constituents of the oil.

Chemotypes, also known as *chemovars*, is where two plants look identical and cannot be separated out into subspecies, but there are differences between them. These differences exist in the chemical constituents and aroma of the plants. Sometimes the common name of the oil will reflect their chemotype.

**Odor and Viscosity of Essential Oils**

Essential oils have the properties of odor and viscosity. *Viscosity* refers to the thickness of the essential oil from thin to thick. Thin essential oils tend to evaporate quickly from a blend, thicker oils tend to have odors that last longer and linger on the body for a longer period of time.

## The Families of Odor

| Family | Scent | Viscosity | Essential Oils |
|---|---|---|---|
| Citrus | Sweet, uplifting | Thin | Bergamot, grapefruit, lemon, lime, orange, tangerine, etc. |
| Floral | Sweet, euphoric | Thin to Medium | Chamomile, geranium, rose, jasmine, lavender, neroli |
| Herbaceous | Green, mossy | Thin to Medium | Basil, clary sage, hyssop, marjoram, melissa, rosemary |
| Woody | Earthy, Smokey | Thin to Medium | Cedarwood, cinnamon, cypress, juniper berry, pine, sandalwood, spruce |
| Spicy | Pungent | Medium to Thick | Aniseed, black pepper, cardamom, cinnamon, coriander, cumin, ginger, nutmeg |
| Resinous | Resinous | Thick | Benzoin, elmi, frankincense, myrrh |
| Camphoaceous | Minty, Earthy | Thin to Medium | Cajeput, eucalyptus, tea tree, peppermint, rosemary, tea |
| Earthy | Sweet Herbaceous | Medium | Angelica, patchouli, valerian, vetiver |

You may blend together essential oils from the same family as listed above.

**Chapter Four**
**Methods of Extraction**

There are several ways that essential oils are produced. Below is a list with brief description of each method currently in use today:

**Distillation Processes**

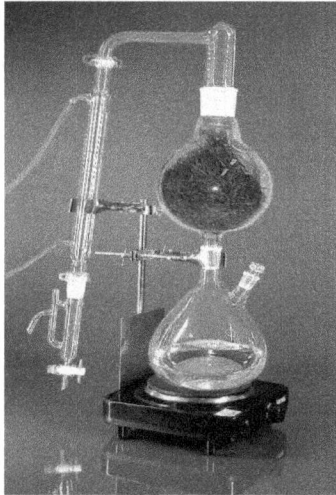

## Hydro Distillation

Process of combining the plant material with water kept in the distillation unit. The unit is heated and essential oil is released into steam droplets that rise and are captured and bottled. This method of distillation is a more watered down method of distillation than steam distillation.

## Steam Distillation

Here, the plant material is stored in a separate compartment away from the tank of water. As the steam is produced in a boiler it is passed through the plant stored outside the tank. The steam comes from the bottom of the tank. Water vapor comes off the plant and carries the essential oil which is caught, cooled and bottled.

### Water or Hydro diffusion
Water diffusion is very similar to steam distillation with one difference, the steam comes from the top onto the botanical material. The condensation of the oil (along with the steam) is hel din place by a grill. In this method, higher oil yields of oils are possible, shorter manufacturing time and less steam is used.

### Solvents
Some flowers used to make essential oils contain too little of the volatile oil or are too delicate to undergo expression or the high heat used in steam distillation. For these flowers, a solvent is used to extract the oils. There are many different kinds of solvents that can be used such as petroleum ether, methanol, ethanol or hexane.

### Concretes
Extracts using hexane and other hydrophobic solvents. Concretes are a mixture of essential oil, waxes, resins and other plant material.

### Absolutes
what is left behind when the alcohol used to extract the essential oil is evaporated. The solvent often used in this process is ethyl alcohol. Plant material is soaked in a solvent (organic chemical like hexane). The mixture of plant material and solvent is called a concrete. Later, the oil is separated from the concrete by using alcohol. This method is often used by perfumeries. The essential oil of Jasmine, Rose and Mimosa is created by this method.

### Florasols
A refrigerant used to replace Freon and also used to extract essential oils at below room temperature to keep degradation of the oils.

### Carbon Dioxide
This process will extract both the waxes and the essential oil that make up the concrete and then process it with liquid carbon dioxide, which will separate the wax from the essential oil at a low temperature to prevent the decomposition and denaturing of compounds. This is a process often used for making decaffeinate coffee.

## Cold Press Extraction (Expression)

This method is the most popular in obtaining citrus oils and is obtained from the rind or peel. This process is also known as scarification. You can accomplish this yourself by placing the plant material between two sheets of glass and placing it out in the hot sun. Droplets of oil with form on the glass-this is the essential oil.

## Carbon Dioxide Extraction

This is a relatively new method of extracting essential oils where $CO_2$ is used to extract the essential oil. This is a very expensive method and is **often used to create essential oils of frankincense and myrrh.**

## Hydrosols

Hydrosols are created during the distillation process. When the vapor is released during the distillation process, it mixes with the steam and then separates once cooled. This separation creates the essential oil and the hydrosol. When created from flowers, hydrosols are sometimes called floral water. Unlike oils, hydrosols cannot be synthetically **manufactured in the lab.**

## Enfleurage

Enfleurage is the process if placing flowers in a vat of odorless and purified solid fats or oils. The fats/oils absorb the essential oil from the plant material. This method is very time consuming but is much like making an infusion with herbs. (generally 2 weeks).

## Hydrosols

Hydrosols are also known as *floral water* and *herbal distillates*. Some see hydrosols as by products from the distillation process or as waste products. So, during the distillation process, there are actually two separate and unique products being created: the essential oil and the hydrosol, or hydrolate.

How this occurs is that during the distillation process, the steam mixes with the plant material and become water and oil. During the cooling process, the water and oil separate creating the essential oil and the hydrolate.

The hydrolate is more than just water; it is water that contains molecules from the plant material and some of the benefits from its mother plant material. Hydrosols are more subtle than essential oils and act more homeopathic. Some popular hydrolates include rose, lavender, and orange.

Since hydrosols still contain some plant material, they must still be handled carefully by either adding a preservative, an alcohol, or kept refrigerated and used quickly. Be sure that the producer of the hydrosol you purchase understands this or you may risk bacterial growth within your product, especially if you are purchasing from someone making oils at their home and may not be well educated in the chemical processes of by-products.

Since there are less chemicals and additives in hydrosols, the essential oil used in these products is much milder and safer. Hydrosols are used primarily in skin care as a body spray, in creams and masks. They can be used in eye inflammations, facial toners, room sprays, astringents (like Witch hazel), cosmetics and toiletries.

**Chapter Five**
**Chemistry**

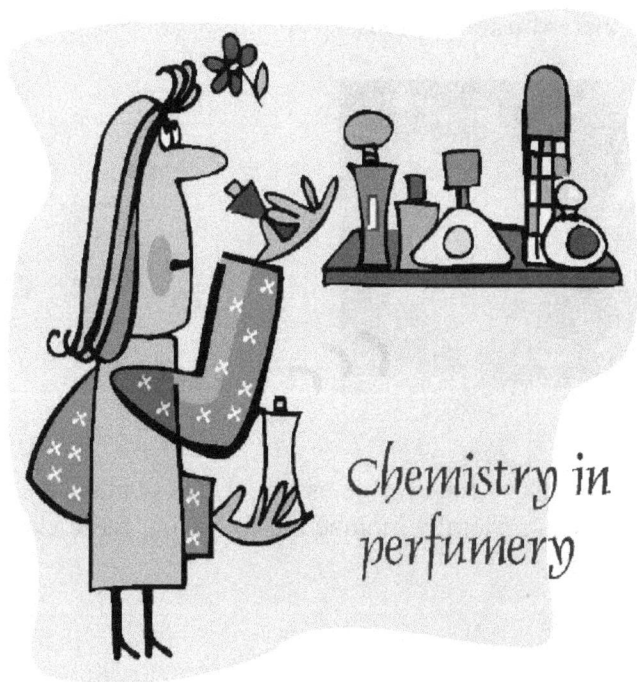

Chemistry in perfumery

In this chapter, we will cover the following information:

Atoms and Molecules
Hydrocarbons
Monoterpenes
Diterpenes
Sesquiterpenes
Alcohols
Phenols
Esters
Ketones
Acids
Aldehydes
Coumarins
Oxides

**Atoms and Molecules**

Atoms are considered the building blocks of live and are the basic components of all substances. Atoms are the smallest unit that exists in a stable form. Each atom consists of a nucleus that is made up of protons and neutrons that orbit the nucleus.

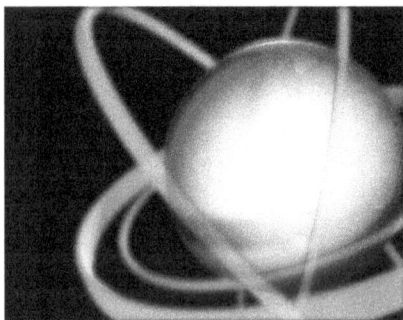

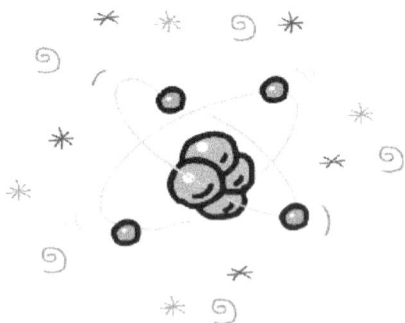

The molecular structures of essential oils contain the elements of life. These elements generally include the following basic elements:
1. carbon (C)
2. hydrogen (H)
3. oxygen (O)

Small amounts of sulphur and nitrogen can also be found at times. When talking about the Chemistry of essential oils, we are talking about the collection of chemical compounds that make up the plant. Below is an example on an essential a-amino acid.

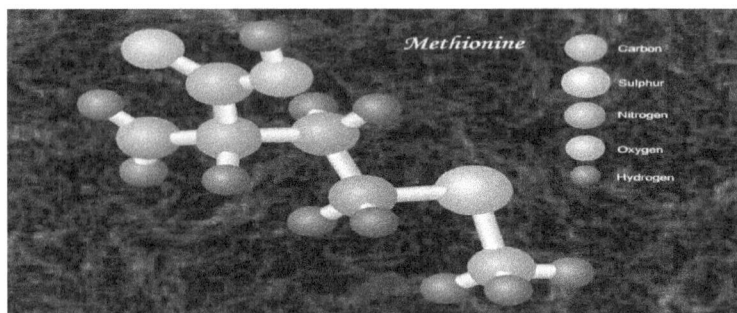

Methionine
Carbon
Sulphur
Nitrogen
Oxygen
Hydrogen

Atoms attract and join with other atoms to stabilize themselves. When atoms come together, they form molecules. Molecules, therefore, are considered compounds because they are made up of more than one element. The type of molecule it becomes is based on the arrangements, number and nature of the atoms that have come together. Almost all molecules that make up essential oils are made from carbon, oxygen and hydrogen. The most often occurring formations are isoprene units which consist of aliphatic chains and aromatic rings.

When we look at organic chemistry, we are looking at carbon based units. Carbon has four chemical bonds that connect it to other carbon atoms where they can form chains and rings. These structures are represented with the letter 'C' to represent carbon, the letter 'O' to represent oxygen, the letter 'H' for hydrogen and 'N' for nitrogen. The bonds between the atoms are presented by a dash.

**Examples of common bonds:**

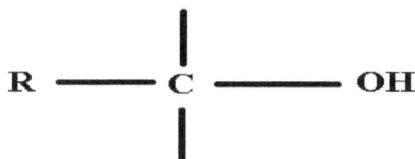

**Alcohol**

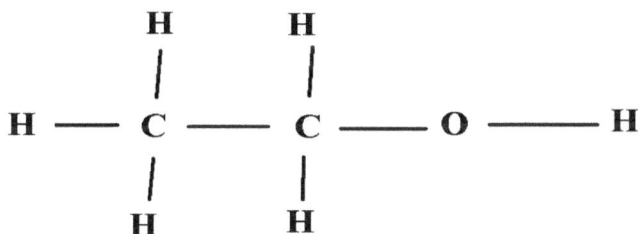

**Ethanol**

**Propanol**

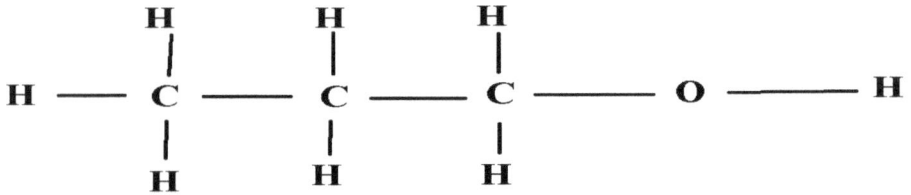

**Hydrocarbons**

Aliphatic chains are also known as terpenes and are present in the majority of essential oils. Terpenes are slightly stimulating, may cause skin sensitivity and are antiseptic in nature.

Monoterpene-(when two isoprene units come together).
Sesquiterpene-(when three isoprene units come together).
Diterpene-(when four isoprene units come togeher).

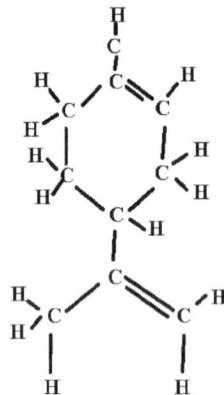

**Monoterpene**

**Terpenes and Essential Oils**

**Monoterpene**-Antibacerial, volatile, highly fragrant, analgesic, and antiseptic. Includes citrus, nutmeg, angelic, pine, fir, spruce and black pepper

**Sesquiterpene**-Anti-inflammatory, hypotensive and sedative. Essential oils in this: Ginger, patchouli, german chamomile, vetiver, sandalwood, ylang ylang

**Diterpene**- Horomone balancing, antifungal, antiviral. An essential oil in this group is carrot seed.

**The two main groups of compounds**
Terpenoids
Phenylpropanoids

**Terpenoids**-formed along the mevalonate pathway in the plant. This is where the essential oil components are made. These compounds have molecules based on the isoprene unit-5 carbon atoms. These compounds join together to create molecules with 10, 15, or 20 carbon atoms-all multiples of 5. Terpenoids are sometimes called *aliphatic compounds*. These compounds end in "ene" such as lemon (limonene) and juniper (a-terpinene/y-terpinene).

Hemiterpenes=5 carbon atoms
Monoterpenes=10 carbon atoms
Sesquiterpenes=15 carbon atoms
Diterpene=20 carbon atoms
Triterpenes=30 carbon atoms
Tetraterpenese=40 carbon atoms

The aromatic rings are associated with Phenylpropanoids. Rings occur when six or more carbon atoms join together. These rings attract the same types of atoms with similar chemical components. The formation of aromatic rings happens when six carbon atoms join together in a ring, as opposed to a straight or branched chain. Aromatic rings can attract the same types of atom groups as aliphatic chains to create similar chemical components. The main difference is aromatic rings can form phenols but they cannot form alcohols.

**Phenylpropanoids**-a smaller group of compounds from the Terpenoids. This group is formed along the shikimate pathway. Their molecules are based on the phenyl ring-6 carbon atoms.

**Alcohols**-Regarded as non-toxic and uplifting. Recognized for their antiseptic, anti-bacterial and anti-viral properties. Stimulates the immune system, general tonic, and diuretic. The following are components of terpene alcohol:

> Citronellol-eucalyptus, geranium, lemon, rose
> Farnesol-chamomile
> Geraniol-garanium, palmarosa
> Linalol-lavender, rosewood

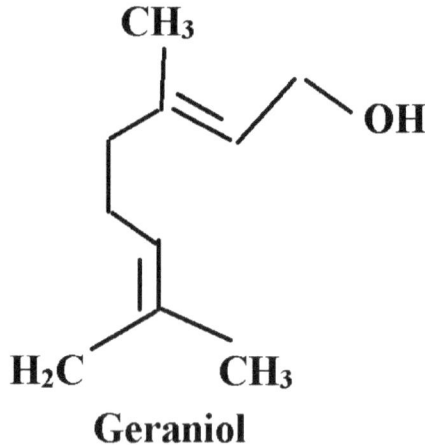

**Geraniol**

The following are components of sesquiterpene alcohol that are anti-bacterial, anti-inflammatory, anti-mycotic and ulcer-protective:

> **Bisabolol**-chamomile oils

**Phenols**-Also called, **carbolic acid**, phenols is the 'fragrance' of an essential oil. Regarded as anti-bacterial, anti-oxidant, antiseptic and stimulating. Phenols are stimulating and aggressive in their effects against infection. May irritate the skin or mucus membranes. Use in small doses for short periods of time.

Phenols whose name ends in 'ol' are part of the alcohol functional group and is used in pain relief. An example would be eugenol in clove bud to relieve tooth pain.

Eugenol-cinnamon and clove

Thymol-thyme

Carvacrol-oregano and savory

Methyl eugenol-basil, bay leaf, cinnamon, clove oi, nutmeg

Methyl chavicol-anise, basil, bay, fennel, tarragon

Safrole-basil, black pepper, cinnamon, nutmeg

Myristicin-dill, parsley

Apiol-dill, fennel, parsley

## Naturally occurring phenol

| Estradiol | estrogen - hormones |
|---|---|
| Dopamine | natural neurotransmitters |
| Adrenaline | natural neurotransmitters |
| Eugenol | clove essential oil |
| Methyl salicylate | the major constituent of the essential oil of wintergreen |
| Salicylic acid | precursor compound to Aspirin |
| Serotonin | natural neurotransmitters |
| Thymol | thyme; an antiseptic that is used in mouthwashes |
| Sesamol | a naturally occuring compound found in sesame seeds |

**Esters**-These are compounds that result from the condensation of an alcohol with an acid and are common in essential oils. Fruit-like odor. Anti-fungal, calming and relaxing. Below is only a sample of some esters and their essential oil connections:

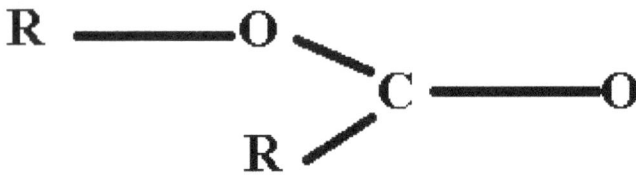

**Esters**

| Ester Name | Odor or occurrence |
|---|---|
| Allyl hexanoate | pineapple |
| Benzyl acetate | jasmine |
| Bornyl acetate | pine |
| Ethyl cinnamate | cinnamon |
| Geranyl acetate | geranium |
| Isopropyl acetate | fruity |
| Linalyl acetate | bergamot, lavender, sage |
| Methyl anthranilate | grape, jasmine |
| Methyl benzoate | fruity, ylang ylang, feijoa |
| Methyl pentanoate (methyl valerate) | flowery |
| Methyl phenylacetate | honey |
| Methyl salicylate (oil of wintergreen) | Modern root beer, wintergreen |
| Nonyl caprylate | orange |
| Octyl acetate | fruity-orange |

**Ketones**-Simple compounds that include many sugars (ketoses). Ketons include the industrial solvent acetone which makes it highly prized in industry. Although not highly toxic in general, some essential oils have been flagged (but not documented) to have caused reaction. These essential oils include mugwort, sage, tansy and wormwood. Ketones are used to help with respiratory issues, cell regeneration, tissue formation and mucous.

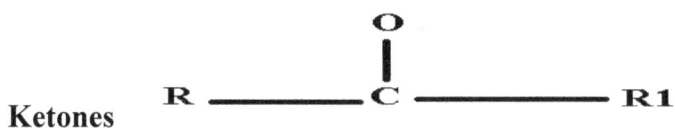

$$R \underline{\hspace{2cm}} \overset{\overset{\textstyle O}{\|}}{C} \underline{\hspace{2cm}} R1$$

**Ketones**

**Ketones**

>    **Thujone**-Highly toxic irritant to the central nervous system. May relieve respiratory issues and stimulate the immune system when inhaled. Sage and wormwood.
>>      asmone-Jasmine
>>      Fenchone-Fennel
>>      Camphor-Used for respiratory issues (Vick's Vapor Rub)
>>      Carvone-caraway and dill
>>      Menthone-geranium, pennyroyal, peppermint
>>      Methyl nonyl-Also known as 2-Undecanone. Clove and rue oils.

7.) **Acids**-Chemical substances that are characterized by a sour taste, ability to turn blue litmus red, and reacts with bases and certain metals to form salts.
>>      Phosphoric acid-production of phosphate fertilizers, cola drinks
>>      Sulfuric acid-dissolves zinc oxide to product zine
>>      Nitric acid-reacts with ammonia to produce a fertilizer
>>      Carboxylic acids-used with alcohols to produce esters
>>      Acetic acid-vinegar
>>      Carbonic acid-cola drinks, soda, maintains pH equilibrium in the body
>>      Citric acid-preservative in sauces and pickles, citrus fruits, lemon and oranges
>>      Tartaric acid-tamarind and unripened mangoes
>>      Oxalic acid-carambola, rhubarb, spinach and tomatoes
>>      Ascorbic acid-Vitamin C. Found in amla, citrus fruits, guava and lemon

Acetylsalicylic acid-Aspirin. Used to reduce fevers and as an analgesic.

Hydrochloric acid-present in stomach and aids in digestion by breaking down food.

Amino acids-helps to synthesis proteins needed for growth and repair of body tissues.

Fatty acids-required for growth and repair of body tissues

Nucleic acids-helps manufacture DNA and RNA.

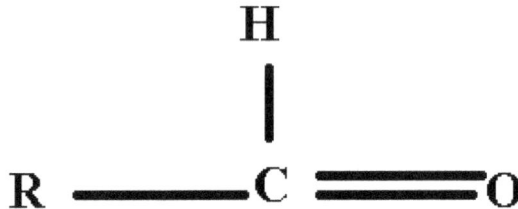

**Aldehydes**

8.)**Aldehydes**-Characterized by the group containing carbon, hydrogen and oxygen known as C-H-O. Most sugars are derivatives of aldehydes. Aldehydes are anti-infectious, photosensitive, calming and sedative on the central nervous system (CNS). May be applied topically or via inhalation.

Citral- antiseptic and anti-viral. Melissa oil.

Citronellal-citronella, lavender, lemongrass, lemon, lemon-scented eucalyptus, mandarin, melissa, myrrh.

Benzaldehyde-almonds, apricots, apples, cherry kernels

Cinnamaldehyde-cinnamon bark, powdered cinnamon

Cuminic aldehyde-cumin

Perillaldehyde-perilla

9.) **Coumarins**-'tonka bean.' Analgesic, antiseptic, Anti-arrhythmia, anti-hypertension, anti-HIV, anti-inflammatory, anti-tumor, anti-osteoporosis. Used to treat lymphedema, asthma, autoimmune deficiency, bone loss, inflammation, appetite suppressant, and pain.

First synthesized in 1868, coumarin is used in the pharmaceutical industry as an anticoagulant similar to dicoumarol or the warfarin (Coumadin). Also used as a edema modifier to allow for the body to reabsorb edematous fluids faster. Coumarin is found naturally in the following plants and extracts:

cassia cinnamon (*Cinnamomum cassia*)
deertongue (*Dichanthelium clandestinum*)
*Justicia pectoralis* extract
mullein (*Verbascum* spp.)
sweet-clover (*Melilotus* ssp.)
sweet grass (*Hierochloe odorata*)
sweet woodruff (*Galium odoratum*)
tonka bean (*Dipteryx odorata*)
vanilla grass (*Anthoxanthum odoratum*)

Coumarin is hepatoxic (toxic to the liver) in rats and moderately toxic to the liver and kidneys in people. The United States Occupational Safety and Health Administration (OSHA) does not classify coumarin as a carcinogen (causing cancer) for humans.

Coumarin is found in some teas, bakery good, strawberries, apricots, cherries, black currants, alcoholic beverages, perfumery, flavors cigarette tobacco and some pipe tobacco (banned in Germany in tobacco use), and in some mulled wine.

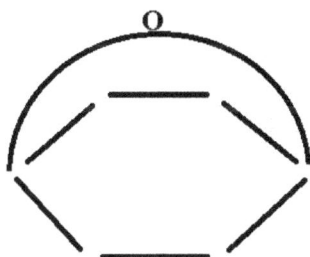

**Oxides**

10.) Oxides-a chemical compound that contains one oxygen atom and at least one other element. Anesthetic, anti-bacterial, Anti-fungal, and antiseptic.

Cineol (or eucalyptol)- basil, cinnamon, eucalyptus, melissa,
ravensara, rosemary
Ascaridol-wormseed oil

| Chemical Group | Characteristics | Safety Issues | Essential Oil |
|---|---|---|---|
| Terpenes -or Monoterpenes 'enes' | Stimulates the immune system. Antiseptic. Volatile, Antibacterial, tonic, antiviral, stimulant | Use with carrier oil, possible skin irritant when oil is old, drying to skin | Citrus and Needle oils, pine, cypress, fir, spruce, juniper berry, peppermint, grapefruit, lemon |
| Sesquiterpenes (strongest odor) | Anti-inflammatory, anti-tumor, liver stimulant, sedative, antiseptic, anti-allergenic, calming | | Roots and Woods, Ginger, patchouli, g. chamomile, vetiver, sandalwood, ylang ylang |
| Monoterpene alcohols | Antimicrobial, sedative, antifungal, antispasmodic, immune supportive | Low toxicity Low irritation | Rose, thyme, geranium, rosewood, citronella peppermint menthol |
| Sequiterpene alchohols end in "ene" | Anti-inflammatory, antispasmodic, sedative, antiseptic | | Sandalwood, nerolina |
| Diterpene (camphorene) | Horomone balancing, antifungal, antiviral | May be purgative | Carrot seed |
| Alcohols | Antiviral, | Non-irritating, | Citronella, |

| | | | |
|---|---|---|---|
| | uplifting, antibacterial, anti-infectious, immune stimulant, energizing | great for children and those with sensitivities | rose, geranium, eucalyptus, rosewood, palmarosa |
| Phenols | Antiseptic, antifungal, anti-bacterial, stimulating | May irritate skin and mucous membrane. Hepatoxic | Aniseed, oregano, cinnamon leaf, clove, fennel seed, thyme CT thhymol |
| Aldehydes End in "al" | Antimicrobial, sedative, hormone balancing | Skin irritant | Melissa, cinnamon, lemongrass, lemon verbena, cinnamon |
| Ketones End in "one" | Antimicrobial, wound healing | Hepatoxic, Neurotoxic | Camphor, Dill, Spearmint |
| Esters | Antispasmodic, sedative, adaplogenic, anti-inflammatory | Safe to use | Roman chamomile, cardamom, lavender, clary sage, wintergreen |
| Lactones (includes coumarins) | Antifungal, antibacterial, mucolytic, expectorant, blood thinner, hypotensive, uplifting, sedative, Coumarins-urinary and coronary dilators | May irritate skin Photosensitivity, Neurotoxic | Inula |

| Ethers | Antispasmodic, carminative, mucolytic, estrogenic effect, antiviral, decongestant, digestive stimulant | Hepatotoxic | Tarragon, basil, fennel, aniseed, clove, basil, tarragon |
|---|---|---|---|
| Oxides | Expectorant, stimulant, antispasmodic | | Eucalyptus, tea tree, spike lavender, rosemary, bay laurel |
| Sesquiterpinols | Anti-inflammatory, hepatonic, tonic, gland stimulant | | Rose, patchouli |
| Diterpinols | Balances the endocrine system | | Clary sage |

**Chapter Six**
**Anatomy, Physiology and the Systems of the Body**

Although two different words, 'anatomy' and 'physiology' they are a very interrelated science. The word *Anatomy* is defined as the study of the structure of an organism and the relationship of its parts. This was mostly discovered by dissecting components of the human body and studying it. The word *Physiology* is the study of the <u>functions</u> of living organisms and theirs parts. Organisms refer to a living thing, an organization of sorts.

There is a set of levels when we look at how our body is organized. We begin with the bottom of the inverted pyramid with the atom. The *atom* is made up of carbon, hydrogen, oxygen and nitrogen. Next is the molecule. *Molecules* are made up of sugars, proteins and water. The atom and molecule are so small that they must be seen through a microscope. This is often referred to as the *chemical level* of organization. They form the cells of the body. The *cell* is considered the smallest 'living' unit in our body. Cells form some specific functions (such as heart cells, nerve cells, muscle cells and epithelial cells).

When many cells come together they can form *tissues* in the body. An example of this would be epithelial tissue, nervous tissue, muscle tissue and connective tissue. Muscle tissue produces movement by contacting and shortening. Epithelial tissue is found throughout the body as lining for internal organs or in the epidermis of the skin. Connective tissue is the ligaments, tendons, bone and cartilage the supports and protects the body structure. Nervous tissue allows electrical impulses to pass between the brain and the rest of the body.

Tissues come together to create *organs* that perform specific functions such as lung, brain, stomach, kidney, etc. When several organs combine together it is called an *organ system*. An organ system works to perform very specific functions. For example, if you would take a look at the digestive system, you will see that it would include such organs as the mouth, tongue, lips, gall bladder, pharynx, parotid gland, salivary glands, spleen, rectum, cecum, stomach, liver, pancreas, small and large intestines, colon, esophagus, etc.

Each organ works together to ingest (take food in to the mouth), digest (break down food in to small molecules), absorb food. (take the nutrients from the food and put in to the blood stream), and then to eliminate it (to remove waste products).

As you can see, there are many activities that must come together for a body system to function properly and successfully. This is why when we look at using essential oils on a person that we must take a look at the entire body system involved in the issue.

In this way, we become better Aromatherapists and better able to help others with their issue. So, we are not just treating a single ailment, which of course we can do at times, but for chronic issues, we must look at the entire body system. It is this organ system that we will now take a look at in this manual.

**These are the systems of the body:**
   **The Limbic System**
   **The Olfactory System**
   **The Nervous System**
   **The Respiratory System**
   **The Integumentary System**
   **The Endocrine (Glandular)**
   **The Circulatory System (Cardiovascular)**
   **The Digestive System**
   **The Lymphatic System**
   **The Musculoskeletal System**
   **The Immune System**
   **The Genita-urinary System**
   **The Reproductive System**


**Homeostasis**
   As a therapist, we are always trying to our client's body back to a system of homeostasis. *Homeostasis* is the relative constancy of the internal environment. It is a balance within the body. This is why it is important for the body to maintain the right temperature, salt content, acid level (pH levels), oxygen concentrate, fluid volume and pressure must all remain within certain limits.

One of the ways that the body can control the systems of the body is by either a positive or negative feedback loop. In the *negative feedback* loop, one day you feel a sudden chill in the air and your body temperature decreases which activates the cold receptors of your body that sends the message to your brain that you are feeling cold. Your body responds by increasing your breathing to bring more oxygen in to your body to help feed your muscles so that they can continue to work to increase your body temperature back to normal. A fever is another example of a negative feedback loop in which the temperature of the body raises in order to 'burn' off the pathogen. Negative feedback loops, regardless of its name, is the most common way our body has as keeping the body in homeostasis. In a *positive feedback* loop, the action of the body is stimulatory. So, instead of challenging the changes in the internal environment, the body responds in a different way and actually amplifies the action. This is seen in giving birth. The body will cause the contractions of the uterus to increase in order to force the baby out of the womb. So in the positive loop, the body works with the action.

**The Limbic System**

The Limbic System, also called the paleomammalian brain, is part of the autonomic nervous system (ANS). This system is sometimes called the emotional brain because this is where the emotions can produce changes in the functions of the body. Emotions can cause the body to perform muscle contractions, glands to secrete, cardiac muscles to contract and hands to sweat. The limbic system is concerned with the sense of smell (olfaction), emotion, behavior, motivation, and long-term memory storage.

Why is knowledge of the limbic system important? It is important because it can affect your client's response to the use of essential oils. Even though you may think that a certain essential oil should have a specific reaction with your client, it may not have that reaction due to an emotion that the client has attached to that aroma. If a client has a negative memory to the smell of lavender, then you using lavender on them with cause a negative reaction. This is why it is important to make sure that the client does not have any aversion to certain essential oils.

This can be handled with the client intake form where the client can write down any essential oils that they do not like. This can also be done in the interview process where you can ask your client about certain essential oils that you are planning on using for them.

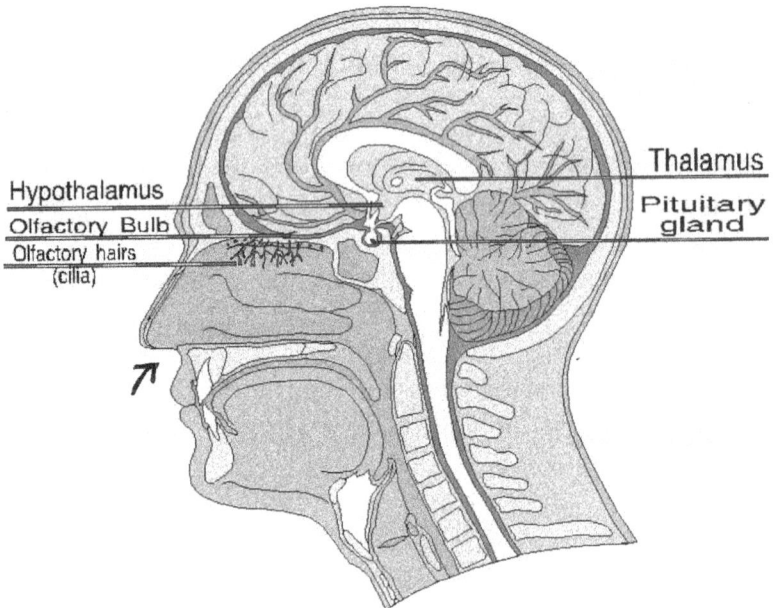

**The Olfactory System**

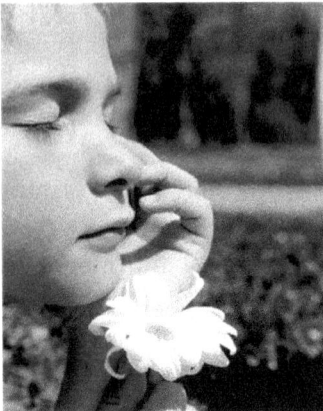

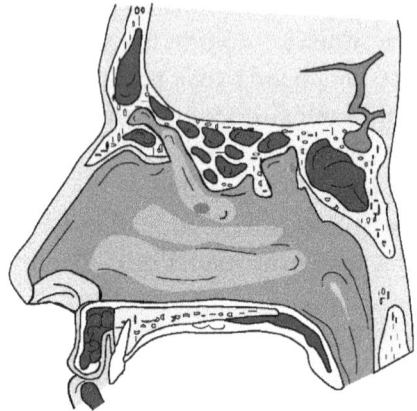

*Olfaction* is how the sense of smell works. It is associated with both the nervous system and the respiratory system. The sense of smell is one of the sensory receptors of our body. Along with the sense of smell we have the following senses: sense of sight (eyes), hearing and balance (ears), and tasting (taste buds). There are other receptors too such as pain receptors that respond to physical damage or injury and thermoreceptors that respond to changes in temperature.

The *olfactory receptors* are located in the small area of epithelial tissue in the upper part of the nasal cavity. These receptors can become very fatigued quickly and after a while they will not be able to sense the odor. This is why we have to 'cleanse our palate' so to speak when we are working with essential oils over a period of time. We can accomplish this by sniffing a container of coffee beans.

Olfactory receptors degenerate over time due to environmental pollutants, smoking and aging. Many older adults suffer from depression with the loss of smell and begin to isolate themselves from other. So, how does the sense of smell work?

With every breath that we take aroma molecules travel a pathway from our nostrils to our brain. This happen thanks in part to a thin layer of sticky mucus that lies at the top of the nose in the epithelium tissue.

Essential oil molecules dissolve in the epithelium tissue and it is then picked up by specialized hair-like receptor cells called *cilia*. From the cilia, the molecules travel to the *olfactory bulb*, the primary organ of smell. This bulb is made up of nervous tissue and contains the only neurons in the body to replace themselves regularly (every 60 days).

When we inhale essential oil molecules, a nerve signal in the form of an electrical impulse is sent to the olfactory bulb which process the information and sends it along to the olfactory tract (a bundle of nerve fibers) to the olfactory cortex, and then to the limbic system. The limbic system is a collection of structures that include the thalamus, the hypothalamus and the amygdale.

The hypothalamus is considered the 'master gland' of the endocrine system and it responsible for regulating several systems of the body such as heart beat, body temperature, hunger, thirst, blood sugar, growth, sleeping, emotions, and more.

Our nose responds in less than 1 second to an odor. Our sense of smell is the only sense that does not need to go through the spinal cord or digestive tract in order to be processed-it can go directly to the brain. The sense of taste is limited to salty, bitter, pungent, astringent, sweet and sour. Our nose can detect approximately 10,000 odors.

About 2 million people in the United States have NO sense of smell. This disorder is called anosmia. A serious head injury can cause anosmia. Most likely this results in damage to the olfactory nerves as they enter the olfactory bulb. It is also possible that damage of the frontal lobes caused by a tumor or surgery can cause anosmia. Elderly people often have a reduced sense of smell.

Researchers Jason Castro from Bates College, Chakra Chennubhotla from the University of Pittsburgh, and Arvind Ramanathan from Oak Ridge National Laboratory published an article in the September 18, 2013 journal *PLOS ONE,* where they identified 10 categories of basic odor qualities.

**These are as follows:**
> **fragrant**
> **woody/resinous**
> **fruity (non-citrus)**
> **chemical**
> **minty/peppermint**
> **sweet**
> **popcorn**
> **lemon**
> **pungent**
> **decayed**

## The Nervous System

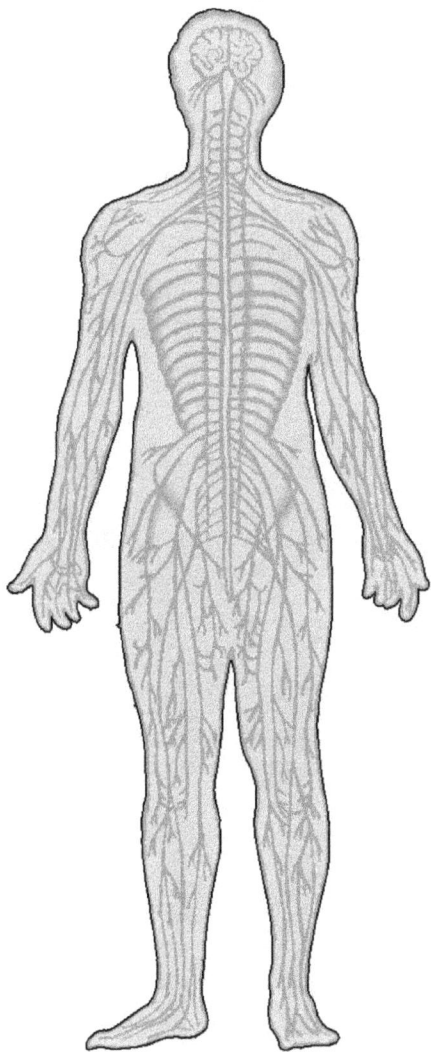

The Nervous System monitors the changes happening inside of the body and reacts to them through electrical impulses between neurons. It does this by receiving information from internal and external sensory receptors and then acting on that information through the muscular and glandular functions of the body.

The nervous system in subdivided in to three parts: the central nervous system (CNS), the peripheral nervous system (PNS), and the autonomic nervous system (ANS). Since the brain and spinal cords make up the midline of the body it is easier to remember them as the central nervous system. The peripheral nervous system consists of the cranial and spinal nerves and is responsible for keeping the body in a state of homeostasis. The autonomic nervous system consists of involuntary functions of the body such as regulating your heart rate, contractions of the stomach while you are eating, etc. These are things that just happen without you concentrating on them or commanding them to happen.

The nervous system has two types of cells called *neurons,* or nerve cells, and *glia,* otherwise known as support cells. There are three types of neurons that transmit impulses. They are the sensory, motor and interneurons.

The sensory neurons transmits impulses directly to the brain and spinal cord (afferent neurons) while the motor neurons transmit impulses away from the brain and spinal cord to the muscle and glandular epithelial tissue (efferent neurons). The interneurons transmit impulses from the sensory neurons to the motor neurons (central neurons).

*Glia,* or neuroglia, is supporting cells. Their job is to hold the functioning neurons together and to protect them. These cells also regulate neuron function.

A *nerve* is a group of peripheral nerve fibers (*axons*) that are bundled together like strands of a cable. A bundle of axons in the central nervous system is called a *tract.* Nerve impulses can travel over trillions of routs called neuron pathways. One such route is called the reflex arc. The response to impulse conduction over a reflex arc is called a *reflex.* The reflex ars it consists of a sensory neuron and a motor neuron. It is responsible for the knee-jerk reflex response that we all know too well.

A *synapse* is the space the separates the axon ending of one neuron from the dendrites of another neuron. The nerve impulse stops at the synapse. It is here that transmission between one neuron to the next occurs. *Neurotransmitters* are chemicals by which neurons communicate. There are least 30 different compounds that have been identified as neurotransmitters that assist, stimulate or inhibit other neurons. These chemicals include dopamine, endorphins, serotonin, etc.

# NERVOUS SYSTEM
Cerebral Hemispheres

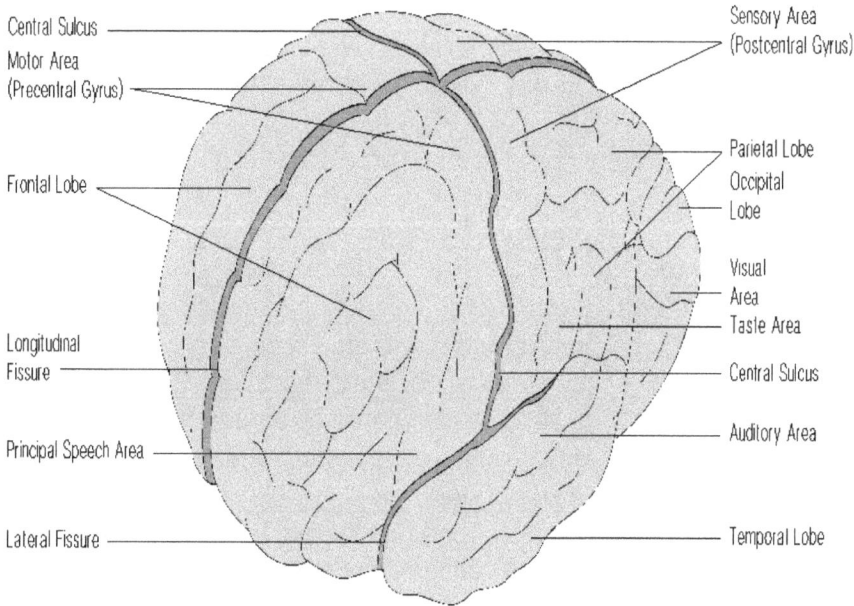

Central Sulcus

Motor Area
(Precentral Gyrus)

Frontal Lobe

Longitudinal
Fissure

Principal Speech Area

Lateral Fissure

Sensory Area
(Postcentral Gyrus)

Parietal Lobe
Occipital
Lobe

Visual
Area
Taste Area

Central Sulcus

Auditory Area

Temporal Lobe

Above is a look at the brain and some of the pathways that the neurons are responsible for such as the five senses. Neurons in the hypothalamus make hormones that the pituitary gland secretes into the blood that affect the volume of urine excreted to keep a water balance in the body.

Essential oils have a strong effect on the nervous system through inhalation, as it goes directly to the hypothalamus. Oils that affect this system include those that are neurodepressants, neurostimulants, analgesics and nervines. Oils can help migraine sufferers, MS, epilepsy and Parkinson's disease by using them to reduce client's stress.

Analgesic-pain. nutmeg, lavender, eucalyptus, marjoram, black pepper, ginger

Shingles-geranium, lavender, r. chamomile, nutmeg, helichrysum, tea tree, Melissa, peppermint, bergamot

Bell's Palsy-bay laurel, rosemary, cypress

Migraines and Headaches-peppermint, lemon, lavender, basil

Epilepsy-bitter orange, lavender, r. chamomile, ylang ylang, clary sage, marjoram

Parkinson's Disease-roman chamomile, basil, linden blossom, rose, black spruce, basil, petitgrain, neroli

Multiple Sclerosis-neroli, rose, rosemary, black spruce, pine, ginger

## Common Pathogens

| Disease/Ailment | Description |
|---|---|
| Alzheimer's disease | Progressive, degenerative disease of the brain |
| Bell's palsy | Inflammation of the facial nerve resulting in paralysis of one side of the face |
| Brain tumor | Cranial tumor (could be benign or malignant) |
| Cerebral palsy (CP) | Brain damage causing motor and posture dysfunctions |
| Concussion | Injury to the brain caused by impact |
| Epilepsy | Neurological disorder caused by interference in the brain's electrical impulses |
| Headaches | Moderate to intense pain in the head |
| Meningitis | Bacteria/viral infection of the meninges surrounding the brain and spinal cord |
| Multiple sclerosis (MS) | Chronic autoimmune disease affects the brain/spinal cord |
| Parkinson's disease | Chronic disorder of the nervous system resulting in tremors |
| Shingles | Painful rash erupting along a sensory nerve path |

# The Respiratory System

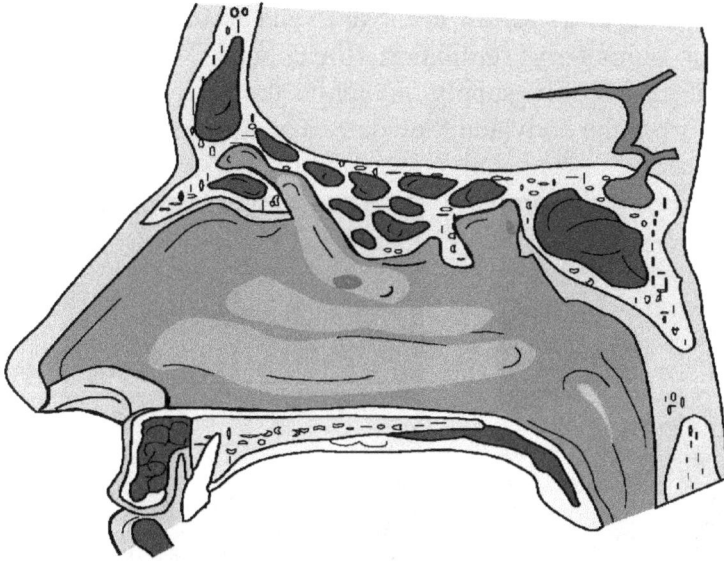

The respiratory system deals with the transportation of oxygen through the body which results in the metabolism of nutrients by inhaling air and oxygen into the lungs. It then expels the carbon dioxide ($CO_2$) as a waste, by-product, through exhalation. The process of inhalation and exhalation is called *respiration.*

Organs of the respiratory system include the nose, lunge, pharynx, larynx, trachea and bronchi. Accessory organs of this system are the diaphragm and intercostal muscles. The organs perform two basic functions: they are air distributors and gas exchangers. They bring oxygen and its vital nutrients into the body and remove carbon dioxide from the body creating a homeostatic mechanism.

There exists an upper and lower respiratory tract. The upper tract includes the nose, pharynx and larynxes while the lower tract contains the trachea, bronchial tree and lungs. The nose moistens and warms the air that we breathe. It contains the sense organs of smell. The Pharynx acts as a passageway for food and liquid to pass. It is also part of the air distribution system as it allows for air to pass through it. The tonsils, part of the phaynx, is a mass of lymphoid tissue that provides immune protection.

The Larynx, also called the Voice Box, is part of the air distribution system as it allows air to move to and from the lungs. The Trachea is also a passageway for air to move to and from the lungs. The lungs provide our pulmonary ventilation (breathing). The lungs have three important functions: they supply oxygen to the body, they remove wastes and toxins from the body and they defend against invasive foreign matter.

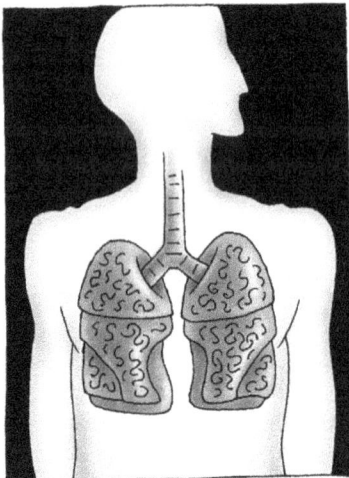

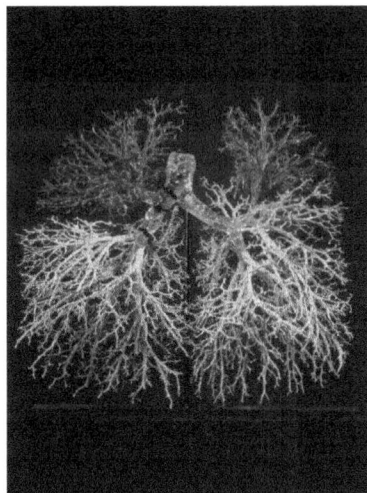

**The pulmonary arteriole and venule, bronchiole**

The Diaphragm contracts and flattens during inhalation and then relaxes during exhalation. The intercostal muscles are located between the ribs and they raise the rib cage when we inhale and relax as we exhale.

*Eupnea* is normal breathing while *hyperventilation* is rapid and deep respirations and h*ypoventilation* is slow and shallow respirations. *Dyspnea* is labored or difficult breathing and *apnea* is when breathing has stopped all together.

Essential oils used for this body system include antispasmodic, decongestants, and expectorants, often used in diffusers, steam inhalations, and facial massages.

Antibacterial-peppermint, lemongrass, cinnamon bark, thyme CT thymol

Antiviral-eucalyptus, ginger, pine, tea tree, Niaouli, ravensara, black pepper

Expectorant-turmeric, eucalyptus, ginger, nutmeg, black spruce, rosemary

Antispasmodic-clary sage, petitgrain, marjoram, basil, tarragon, frankincense

Decongestant-eucalyptus, rosemary, cardamom, spike lavender

## Common Pathogens

| Disease/Ailment | Description |
|---|---|
| Asthma | Chronic inflammatory disease causes swelling in the bronchial tubes or lining of the trachea |
| Bronchitis | Inflammation of a bronchus |
| Bronchogenic carcinoma | Malignant tumor originating in the bronchi. Also called Lung Cancer. |
| Chronic obstructive disease (COPD) | Progressive, chronic groups of pulmonary conditions with obstruction of air through the airways. |
| Common cold | Viral infection that causes nasal congestion, etc.. |
| Croup | Acute respiratory condition with a barking cough |
| Deviated septum | Nasal septum strays from the midline of the nasal cavity |
| Emphysema | Ruptured alveoli in the lungs make breathing difficult |
| Epistaxis | A nosebleed |
| IRDS | Disease characterized by lack of surfactant in the alveoli |
| Laryngitis | Inflammation of the mucous lining of the larynx |
| Pharyngitis | Inflammation or infection of the pharynx |
| Pneumonia | Acute inflammation of the lungs |
| Rhinitis | Inflammation of the nasal mucosa |
| Tuberculosis | Chronic bacillus infection affecting the lungs |

## The Integumentary System (skin)

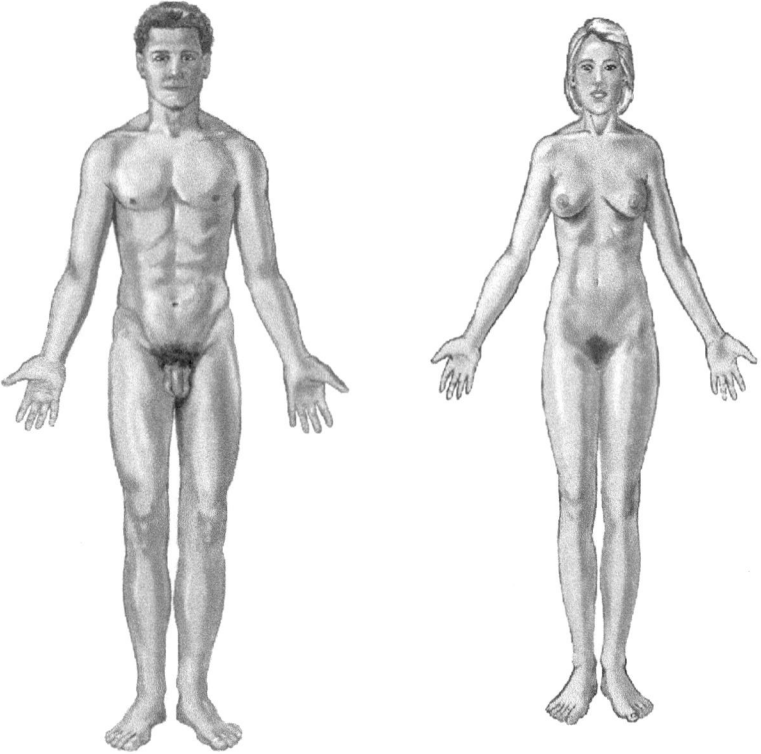

The largest organ of the body, the skin is the body's protection against heat, light, dehydration and pathogens. The skin regulates the heat in the body, secretes perspiration to cool the body and sebum to lubricate the skin, it excretes wastes and absorbs Vitamin D for the body to use.

The skin also has appendages which include the hair, nails and the skin gland. These appendages, along with the skin itself as the principal organ, are all part of the integumentary system. The functions of the integumentary system include:

Protection-The skin forms a barrier to ward against invading and harmful pathogens such as viruses and bacteria. It also protects internal organs from harmful ultraviolet rays.

Regulation-The skin allows us to sweat when we are hot in order to allow evaporation to cool us. Superficial blood vessels constrict to warm us. And a layer of fat (lipids) offers us a layer of insulation.

Sensory reception-The skin has millions of sensory receptors that can detect pain, touch, pressure, temperature, etc. and send these messages to the brain and spinal cord to act on. (Like to remove your hand from a fire).

Secretion-The skin has *sebaceous* glands that secrete oil, sebum, to lubricate the skin. Sweat glands maintain the internal temperature of the body.

## Layers of the skin

**Epidermis-**This is the first layer of the skin and forms the outer membrane. Here a substance called *keratin*, a waterproof material, provides cells with a protective and abrasion-resistant quality.
**Dermis-**This is the middle layer of the skin where you will find the hair follicles, sebaceous and sweat glands, blood vessels, lymph vessels, sensory receptors, nerve and muscle fibers.
**Subcutaneous-**This is the third layer of skin which is formed of fat cells called *lipocytes*. This fat serves as insulation for heat and cold.

**Accessories Organs-**Accessory organs of the skin are the hair, nails, receptors, sweat glands, and sebaceous glands.

## Wound and Tissue Repair

Skin goes through three separate phases in order to accomplish tissue and wound repair. These phases are: inflammation, regeneration and remodeling.

### Common Pathogens

| Disease/Ailment | Description |
|---|---|
| Acne | Inflammatory condition of the sebaceous glands and hair follicles resulting in pimples, cysts, blackheads, etc. |
| Basal cell carcinoma | Cancerous tumor of the epidermis from sun exposure |
| Burns | Injury to skin tissue by heat, fire, chemicals, |

| | etc. |
|---|---|
| Cellulitis | Cute infection and inflammation of the skin |
| Dermatitis | Inflammation of the skin |
| Eczema | Inflammation of the epidermis with red, itchy lesions |
| Folliculitis | Inflammation of the hair follicles with pustules |
| Furnucle | Bacterial infection of a hair follicle with pain. A boil. |
| Gangrene | Tissue necrosis usually due to deficient blood supply |
| Herpes | Small, painful blisters caused by herpes virus |
| Kaposi's sarcoma | Skin cancer often seen in AIDS |
| Malignant melanoma | Skin cancer that spreads to the internal organs |
| Nevus | Pigmented elevated spot on the surface of the skin (mole) |
| Psoriasis | Chronic inflammatory condition with crusty lesions |
| Purpura | Hemorrhages in the skin due to fragile blood vessels |
| Rubella | Contagious viral skin infections with rash and fever |
| Scabies | Contagious skin disease with itching, blisters and pustules |
| Shingles | Rash and pain that erupts along nerve paths of the body |
| Squamous cell carcinoma (SCC) | Epidermal cancer resulting in a crusted nodule that ulcerates and bleeds |
| Tinea | Fungal skin disease with itchy, scaly lesions and rash |
| Urticaria | Skin eruption of pale red itchy wheal. (hives) |
| Vitiligo | Lack of pigment in areas of the skin causing white appearance. Whole body vitiligo is referred to as albino. |
| Warts | Benign growth with rough surface caused by a virus |

Essential oils can be used for scar and wound healing, burns, dermatitis, eczema, psoriasis, and more through topical uses in massage, baths, and compresses.

Anti-inflammatory-lavender, chamomile, tea tree, rose, yarrow

Cicatrizants-lavender, rose, frankincense, g. chamomile, myrrh, helichrysum, neroli

Scars-lavandin, lavender, tea tree, ginger, black pepper, juniper, rosemary

Burns-lavender, g. chamomile, peppermint

Dermatitis and Eczema-mandarin, geranium, palmarosa, rose, calendula

Psoriasis-lavender, german chamomile, rose, palmarosa, calendula, mandarin, helichrysum, neroli, grapefruit, blue cypress

Anti-pruritics-lavender, tea tree, peppermint

Moisturizers-german chamomile, mandarin, sweet orange, rose, geranium, palmarosa

## The Endocrine System

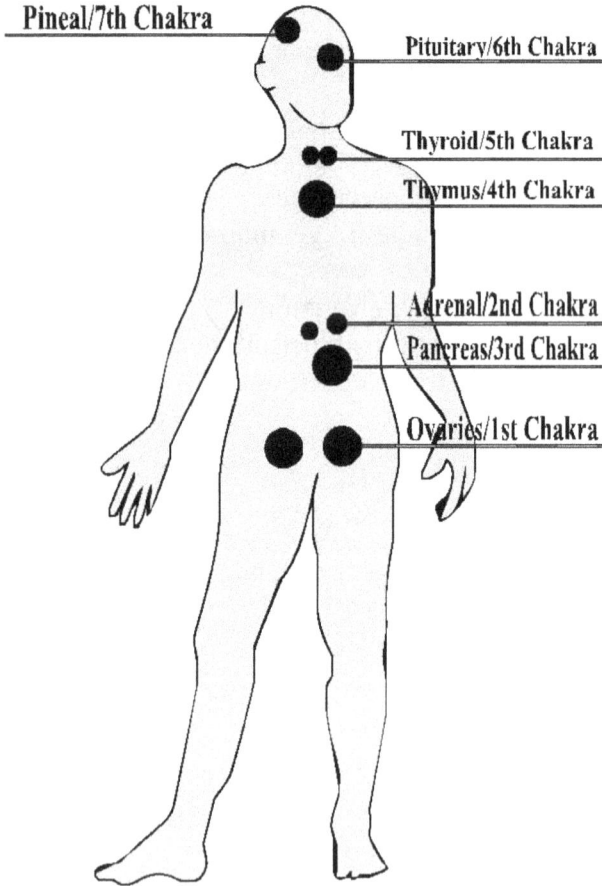

Pineal/7th Chakra

Pituitary/6th Chakra

Thyroid/5th Chakra

Thymus/4th Chakra

Adrenal/2nd Chakra

Pancreas/3rd Chakra

Ovaries/1st Chakra

    The endocrine system is made up of a group of glands known for the hormones that they secrete. The endocrine system secretes hormones and chemical messengers into the blood stream to target specific organs or cells in the body. These hormones regulate growth, sexual function, immune responses, metabolism, development and water and mineral balances in the body.

The glands of the endocrine system are either endocrine glands or exocrine glands. *Endocrine glands* are ductless glands that secrete chemicals known as hormones into intercellular spaces. There are approximately 10 major endocrine glands of the body which includes the hypothalamus, pituitary, pineal, parathyroid, thyroid, thymus, adrenals, pancreatic islets, testes (male) and ovaries (female).

The exocrine glands secrete their products into ducts that empty in to a cavity or on to a surface. Examples of exocrine glands are sweat glands that produce secretions on the surface of the skin and salivary glands that secrete saliva that flows into the mouth. *Hypersecretion* is when a diseased gland produces too much secretion and *hyporsecretion* is when too little hormone is produced.

The major organs of the endocrine system are as follows:

**Pineal**-Secretes melatonin and serotonim

**Pituitary**-Called the 'Master Gland' of the body because this small, bean shaped organ and its secretions regulate all of the endocrine glands. This gland produces the growth hormone, thyroid-stimulating hormone, adrenocorticotropin hormone, prolactin, follicle-stimulating hormone, melacocyte-stimulating hormone, and luteinizing hormones. Also included is the antidiuretic hormone and oxytocin.

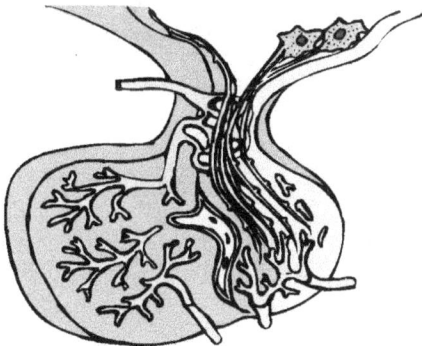

# Pituitary Gland

Thyroid-Secretes thyroxine (T4), Triiodothyronine (T3) and calcitonin.

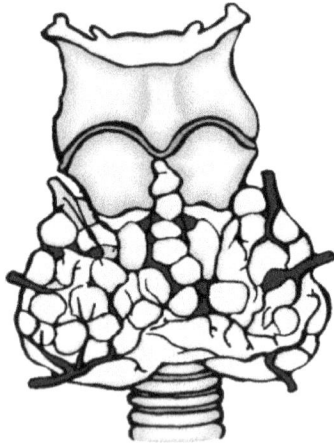

The Thyroid Gland

**Parathyroid**-Secretes parathyroid hormone
**Thymus**-Secretes thymosin
**Adrenal**-Secretes cortisol, corticosterone, aldosterone, testosterone, andosterone, dopamine, epinephrine and norepinephrine
**Pancreas**-Secretes insulin and glucagon

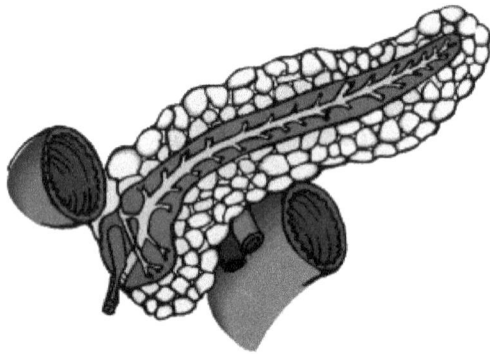

The Pancreas

**Ovaries**-Secretes estrogen and progesterone
**Testes/Gonads**-Secretes testoterone

## Common Pathogens

| Disease/Ailment | Description |
| --- | --- |
| Acromegaly | Hypersecretion of growth hormone. Gigantism. |
| Addison's disease | Hyposecretion of adrenocortical hormone |
| Cushing's disease | Hypersecretion of cortisol in adrenal cortex. Moon face. |
| Diabetes insipidus | Inadequate secretion of antidiuretic hormone (ADH |
| Diabete's mellitus | Not enough insulin produced or body not using hormone |
| Dwarfism | Hyposecretion of growth hormone (GH) |
| Goiter | Enlargement of thyroid gland due to lack of iodine |
| Grave's disease | Hyposecretion of thyroid hormones T3 and T4 |
| Hyperthyroidism | Deficient T3 and T4 in thyroid gland secretions |

Pineal-sandalwood, rosemary
Pituitary-Sage(estrogen and progesterone-testosterone balance), petitgrain, peppermint, citrus oils, lavender, rosemary, sandalwood, ylang ylang,
Thyroid/Parathyroid-spearmint, myrtle, elemi, thyme.
Thymus-myrrh, palmarosa
Adrenal-pine, spruce, lavender, cedar, peppermint, citrus oils, nutmeg, ambrette, rose geranium,
Pancreas-g. chamomile, orange, coriander, dill, cinnamon, and cypress
Ovaries-clary sage, helichrysum, frankincense, geranium, cypress, lavender
Testes/Gonads-r. chamomile, lavender, rosemary

# The Circulatory (Cardiovascular) System

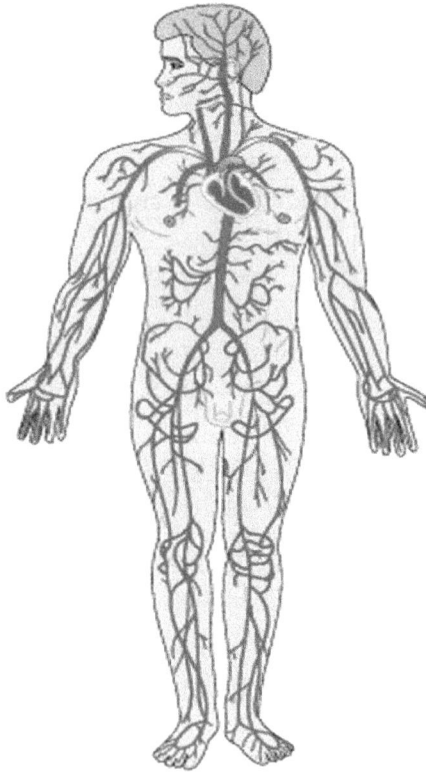

It's the responsibility of the Circulatory (Cardiovascular) System to transport oxygen and nutrients, remove wastes, to regulate the body's temperature, hormone levels and pH of fluids. The heart is the major organ of this system of the body. It contains four chambers, or cavities, that pump and circulate blood through the body and lungs. It weight approximately 9 ounces and is the size of human fist. It is controlled by the autonomic nervous system which means that you don't have to make it pump blood; it does this on its own. It is blood vessels that transports blood away from the heart and back again. There are three major blood vessels: Arteries, veins, and capillaries.

*Arteries* transport blood away from the heart while veins transport blood back to the heart. The largest artery in the body is called the *aorta*. The walls of the arteries expand during the contraction of the heart and relax between the beats of the heart. When you take a pulse, it reflects the rate of the heart.

*Veins* have thin walls and transport blood from tissues and the lungs back to the heart again to become filtered. Veins are generally located closer to the surface of the skin are often used to administer intravenous medications (IV) or when you need to have blood drawn.

The *capillaries* are tiny blood vessels with thin walls that serve as exchange vessels. Capillaries send vital oxygen and nutrients to tissues and receive waste products and carbon dioxide in exchange.

Blood is the life line of the body. It is the fluid that transports oxygen from the lungs, nutrients to the cells, hormones from the endocrine system and protects the body from invasion and infection. Blood regulates the pH levels of the body and balances the electrolytes to insure proper cell functioning.

Deoxygenated blood flows from the heart to the lungs where it receives oxygen. From the lungs, oxygenated blood flows back to the heart and out to the body via the aorta.

Blood pressure is the measurement of the force exerted by blood against the walls of the blood vessel. It is measured in two numbers, one placed over the other. The top number is called the systolic pressure (recorded during ventricular contraction) and the bottom number is called the diastolic pressure (recorded during ventricular relaxation. The top number (systolic) should always be higher than the bottom number (diastolic). A normal blood pressure for adults is calculated at 120/80, but a healthy range is anything between 90/60 to 140/90.

Aromatherapy affects the cardiovascular system by increasing local circulation, reducing clotting, reducing high blood pressure through massage, reducing angina and arrhythmia by relaxing and balancing the cardiovascular system. Varicose veins may be helped with essential oils as will bruising and inflammation.

**Essential Oils for this system:**

Hypotensive-help to lower blood pressure by dilating blood vessels (vasodilation), relaxing the smooth muscle of the vein's walls (vasorelaxation), or increasing parasympathetic nerve activity/decreasing nerve activity. Lavender, celery seed, basil, cedarwood, neroli, spikenard, ylang ylang, geranium

Hypertensive-raises blood pressure. Cyprus, lemon, juniper

Rubefacient-Increases local peripheral circulation. Cinnamon, eucalyptus

Anticoagulant-for people who have risks for blood clots. Basil, cinnamon leaf, helichrysum

Varicose veins-cypress, lemon, geranium, peppermint, juniper, grapefruit, palmarosa, helichrysum

## Common Pathogens

| Disease/Ailment | Description |
|---|---|
| Anemia | Deficiency of red blood cells in the blood |
| Aneurysm | Weakness in artery wall causing a sac to form |
| Angina pectoris | Severe chest pain with constriction around the heart |
| Angioma | Tumor consisting of blood vessels; usually benign |
| Arrhythmia | Irregular heartbeat |
| Arteriosclerosis | Hardening or thickening of the walls of the arteries |
| Arteritis | Inflammation of an artery |
| Atherosclerosis | Buildup of fatty substances on the inner walls of the arteries |
| Cardiomyopathy | Disease that deteriorates the heart muscle |
| Embolism | Obstruction of a blood vessel by a blood clot or object |
| Hypertension | High blood pressure |
| Hypotension | Low blood pressure |
| Ischemia | Lack of blood supply due to an obstruction |
| Leukemia | Cancer of the white blood cells |
| Phlebitis | Inflammation of a vein |
| Spider veins | Superficial network of veins |
| Thrombus | Blood clot within a blood vessel |
| Varicose Veins | Swelling of veins in legs |

# The Digestive System

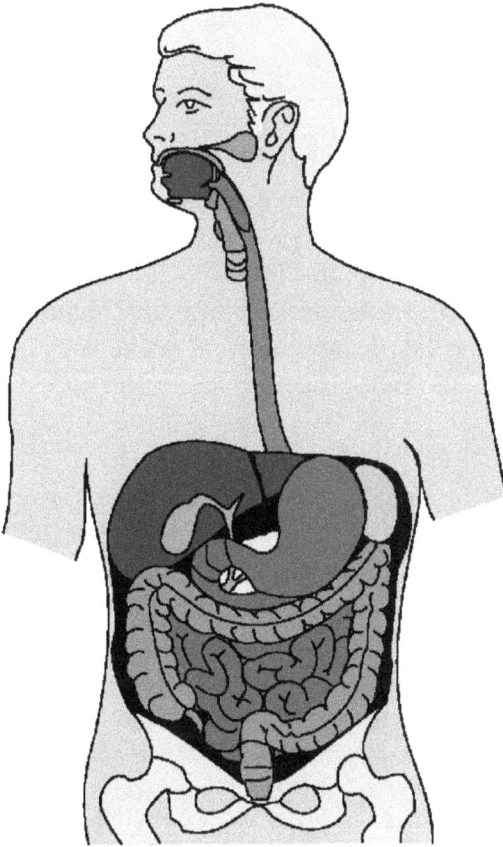

The Digestive System is an irregular hollow tube that provides nutrients, energy, and fuel to the body. Food is taken into the body through a system called *ingestion* and broken down into molecules through a process called *digestion*. These molecules (nutrients) can then be absorbed through the body in a process called *absorption*. The final stage of the digestive system is the removal of leftover waste products through a process called *elimination* in the form of feces.

The main organs of the digestive system are the oral cavity, mouth, pharynx (throat), esophagus, stomach, small and large intestine, cecum, colon, rectum and anal canal. Accessory organs of this system include the teeth, tongue, salivary glands, liver, gallbladder, pancreas and vermiform appendix.

There are several juices and enzymes that are present in the chemical digestion process. These include saliva, gastric juice (pepsin), pancreatic juice (proteases, lipases and amylase) and intestinal enzymes (peptidases, sucrose, lactase, and maltase).

Digestion begins in the oral cavity with the mouth, teeth and salivary glands. In the mouth, food is chewed in a process called *mastication,* by the teeth while the salivary glands secrete saliva to moisten the food and begin the chemical process of breaking down the food. Mastication is the first process in digestion and is completed by the teeth.

The tongue assists in moving the food around and finally swallowing it. The tongue has several taste buds that can identify bitter, sweet, sour and salty flavors. It can also determine temperature, texture and taste thanks to sensory neurons.

The pharynx is the beginning of the tube that leads to the stomach and allows food and liquid to pass through to the esophagus. The epiglottis covers the trachea to prevent food to pass into the airways.

Food continues its journey through the esophagus where wavelike, muscular contractions called *peristalsis*, push the food through the esophagus to the rest of the tract into the saclike, muscular organ called the stomach. In the stomach food is collected and the process of digestion continues and the food moves on to the small intestine.

The longest part of the gastrointestinal tract is the small intestine. Some 20 feet long and 1 inch in diameter, the small intestine begins to absorb the nutrients from the food and liquids it receives. These nutrients are absorbed by the small capillaries that line the walls of the small intestine and are taken to body cells through the circulatory system.

What is left of the food passes on to the large intestine, which is five feet long and 2.5 inches in diameter. Here food and water continues to be absorbed by the body. The bacteria that live in the large intestine contribute to the breakdown of indigestible materials and produce B complex vitamins and Vitamin K which is needed for clotting.

What remains of the food is taken to the rectum where it is stored and compacted. It is then eliminated from the body through the anus in the form of feces.

Essential oils that most influence this body system includes: calming, antispasmodic, digestive stimulants, appetite stimulants or suppressers, and hepatics. These oils can be used in enemas, baths, compresses, rubs, heat applications, and massages.

   Antispasmodic-peppermint, nutmeg, tarragon, Melissa,
         cardamom, basil, sweet orange, rose, roman chamomile
   Digestive stimulant-sage, rosemary, fennel
   Appetite stimulant-cardamon, lemon, peppermint, bergamot,
         fennel, tarragon
   Constipation-fennel, black pepper, marjoram, ginger, sweet
         orange
   IBS-german chamomile, yarrow, lavender, turmeric, helichrysum,
         peppermint, rosemary, cardamom, tarragon, sweet orange


## Common Pathogens

| Disease/Ailment | Description |
|---|---|
| Anorexia | Loss of appetite |
| Anorexia nervosa | Eating disorder involving refusal to eat |
| Appendicitis | Inflammation of the appendix |
| Bulimia | Eating disorder characterized by binging then purging |
| Cholecystitis | Inflammation of the gallbladder caused by gallstones |
| Cirrhosis | Chronic disease of the liver causing liver dysfunction |
| Colorectal cancer | Cancers of the colon |
| Constipation | Difficult or infrequent defecation |
| Crohn's disease | Chronic inflammatory bowel disease affecting the colon |

| Diarrhea | Passing of frequent watery bowel movements |
|---|---|
| Diverticulitis | Inflammation of a diverticulum |
| Diverticulosis | Condition of having diverticula in the intestinal tract |
| Dyspepsia | Indigestion |
| Enteritis | Inflammation of the small intestine |
| Gastritis | Inflammation of the stomach |
| Gastroenteritis | Inflammation of the stomach and small intestine |
| Hemorrhoids | Varicose veins in the rectum |
| Hepatitis | Inflammation of the liver generally due to viral infection |
| Hiatal hernia | Abnormal protrusion in the upper portion of the stomach |
| (IBS) Inflammatory bowel disease | Chronic inflammatory condition with multiple ulcers forming on the mucous membrane of the color. |
| Inguinal hernia | Abnormal protrusion of a portion of the small intestine |
| (IBS) Irritable bowel syndrome | Disturbances in intestinal function from unknown causes. Also called spastic colon. |
| Pancreatic cancer | Cancer of the pancreas |
| Peptic ulcer disease | Ulcer occurring in the lining of the lower esophagus, stomach or duodenum. |
| Polyps | Small tumors attached to the mucous membrane of the colon and/or large intestine. |
| Pyrosis | Painful burning sensation cause by stomach acid. Heartburn. |
| Volvulus | Painful condition where the bowel twists up on itself. |

**The Lymphatic System**

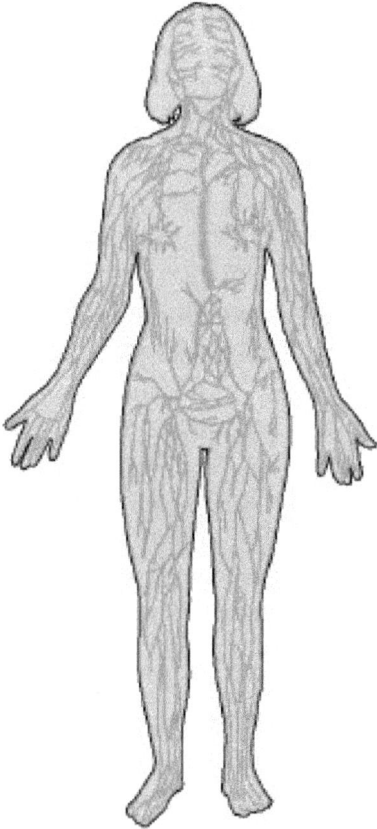

# Lymphatic System

The Lymphatic System consists of lymphatic vessels, nodes, organs, and fluid called *lymph*. The function of this body system is to transport fluid and is vital to the immune system as it traps and destroys pathogens in the body. Parts of the lymphatic system include lymphatic vessels, ducts, nodes, spleen thymus gland and the tonsils.

The lymphatic system is also part of the immune system. Here, this system defends the body against pathogens and foreign invaders. It also removes cells that have become diseased. But the immune system also depends upon many of the tissues and organs of the lymphatic system including:

Intact skin
Secretions (tears and mucus)
White blood cells
Body chemical (hormones and enzymes)
Antibodies

*T lymphocytes*, or T cells, are found in the thymus, a small lymphoid tissue organ in the neck. These cells play a role in the immunity system which we will look at next. The thymus gland is the largest at puberty and weighs approximately an ounce. By the time you reach 60, the gland is about half of its size and by 80 it is gone.

The spleen is the largest lymphoid organ in the body. Even though this organ is protected by the lower ribs, abdominal trauma may cause the spleen to become damaged. The spleen removes bacteria and foreign substances in the blood. It also removes worn-out red blood cells and saves iron found in hemoglobin for later use.

Aromatherapy may help with many disorders of the lymphatic system such as *edema*, an accumulation of blood and fluid, by using oils in a massage. *Cellulite* is a stagnation and accumulation of fluid. Compression and massage can be used to move stagnate fluid through the body

Astringent-tightening effect on tissue (firms tissue)
Diuretic-stimulates the kidneys to produce urine. Grapefruit, lemon, cypress, juniper, fennel, geranium
Hepatic-stimulates the liver. Grapefruit, lemon, cypress, juniper, fennel, geranium
Blood circulatory stimulant-rosemary, black pepper, cinnamon, ginger, juniper
Edema-grapefruit, juniper fennel, german chamomile, rosemary
Cellulite-clove, cinnamon, ginger, peppermint and juniper

**Common Pathogens**

| Disease/Ailment | Description |
|---|---|
| AIDS Aquired Immunodeficiency Syndrome | Disease involving a defect in the cell Syndrome of opportunistic infections |
| Allergy | Response to a common substance in the environment |
| Autoimmune disorder | Defective immune system produces antibodies against itself. |
| Hodgkin's Disease | Cancer of the lymphatic system |
| Lymphadenitis | Inflammation of the lymph nodes (swollen glands) |
| Lymphangioma | Benign mass of lymphatic vessels |
| Lymphodema | Fluid buildup in extremities due to obstruction |
| Lymphoma | Malignant tumor of the lymph nodes and tissues |
| Mononucleosis | Acute infectious disease with abnormal lymphocytes |
| Splenomegaly | Abnormal spleen enlargement |
| Thymoma | Malignant tumor of the thymus gland |

## Musculoskeletal System

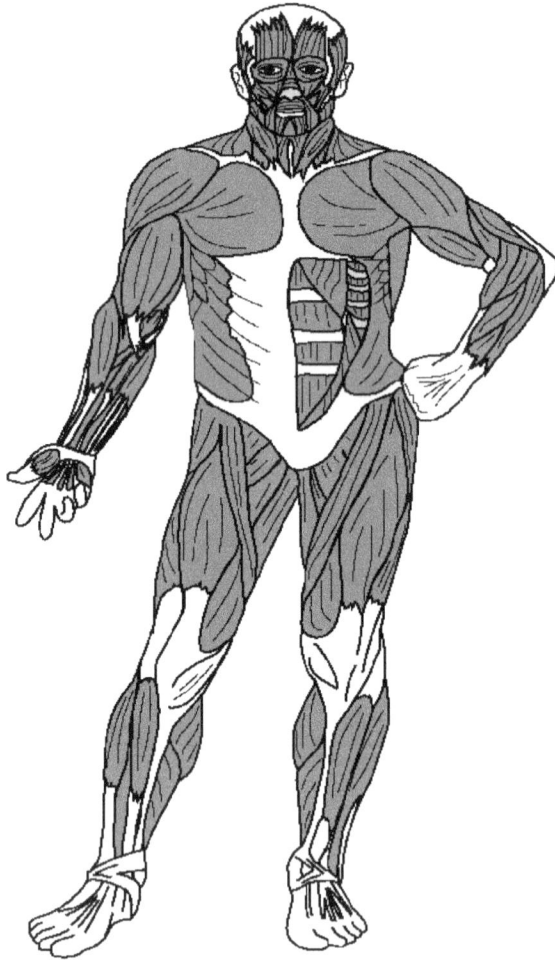

The Musculoskeletal System deals with movement of the body, posture, stability, and holding the bones and joints stable. This system contains the muscles, connective tissues, bones, ligaments, tendons and fascia. There are three major types of muscles: skeletal, smooth and cardiac.

There are hundreds of skeletal muscles in the human body. These muscles are composed of a group of fibers and are held together by connective tissue called *fascia*. Skeletal muscles attach directly or indirectly to bones and overlap joints. These muscles provide for a variety of voluntary body movement by contraction, extension and elasticity.

Smooth muscles are responsible for the involuntary actions of the muscle such as pushing food through the digestive system, uterine contractions, constricting or dilating a blood vessel, etc. They are generally found in the digestive organs, respiratory organs, vascular organs, etc.

Cardiac muscles comprise the wall of the heart and are called *myocardium*. These muscles produce the involuntary actions that cause the heart to pump blood through the chambers and blood vessels. This happens without us thinking about it.

There are many diseases, ailments and disorders that are specifically associated with the muscular system. On the following page is a small list of some of those pathogens.

**Method of Application**

Essential oils can affect the muscles of the body by absorption through the skin, compresses, internally and topically. You can apply (massage or by compresses) essential oils to affected areas of the body to increase circulation, to cool, as an anti-inflammatory, analgesic for pain relief, antispasmodic (for stomach cramping, etc.)

Methods of application for this system include cold and hot compresses for sprains and strains, arthritis joints, aching muscles, cramps and spasms. Baths using essential oils and massaging with essential oils can help with muscles strains and sprains, knotted muscles, Fibromyalgia and for overuse injuries. This includes stress, TMJ, and tension headaches.

Analgesic-bay laurel, eucalyptus, black pepper, chamomile,
      lavender, lavandin, nutmeg, peppermint, sweet birch,
      wintergreen
Anti-inflammatory (*cooling*)-blue cypress, chamomile,
      helichrysum, lavender, palmarosa, sweet birch, turmeric,
      wintergreen, yarrow

Anti-inflammatory (*warming*)-black pepper, clover, cardamom, cumin, ginger, nutmeg

Antispasmodic-basil, black pepper, cardamom, clary sage, lavender, marjoram, petitgrain, r. chamomile

Arthritis-spike lavender, bay laurel, ginger, cardamom

Gout-lavender, peppermint, g. chamomile, helichrysum, yarrow, grapefruit, carrot, juniper

Scleroderma-calendula rose hip, sandalwood, rose, palmarosa, rock rose, geranium

Fibromyalgia-bay laurel, eucalyptus, black pepper, ginger

Cramps and Spasms-marjoram, basil, cardamom, sage, r. chamomile, tarragon

TMJ-wintergreen, marjoram, black pepper, sweet birch, basil, g. chamomile.

Tension Headaches-lavender, basil, rosemary, r. chamomile, peppermint

# Common Pathogens

| Disease/Ailment | Description |
|---|---|
| Adhesion | Built up of layers of fascial tissue |
| Atrophy | Loss of muscle mass/strength due to immobility |
| Bursitis | Inflammation of a bursa |
| Contracture | Shortening of muscle fibers, tendons or fascia |
| Cramps | Involuntary and painful muscle twitch (spasm) |
| Fibromyalgia | Chronic condition of pain and aching muscles-18 points |
| Hernia | Tear in muscle wall that allows an organ to protrude |
| Muscular Dystrophy (MS) | Chronic, genetic diseases causing muscles to degenerate and weaken ending in atrophy |
| Myasthenia gravis | Autoimmune muscle disease causing weakness/fatigue |
| Repetitive Motion Disorder | Damage to joints, muscles, etc. due to repetitive motions. |
| Scar Tissue | Collagen fibers laid down over areas of injury in muscle |
| Spasms | Sudden and violent muscle contraction. A cramp. |
| Sprain | Acute injury to ligaments around joints (whiplash) |
| Strains | Injury or tear in muscle, tendon and attachments to bone |
| Tendinitis | Inflammation of a tendon after repetitive movements |
| Tetanus | Bacterial disease causing locking of the jaw |
| TMJ | Muscle contraction of the jaw |

**The Skeletal System**

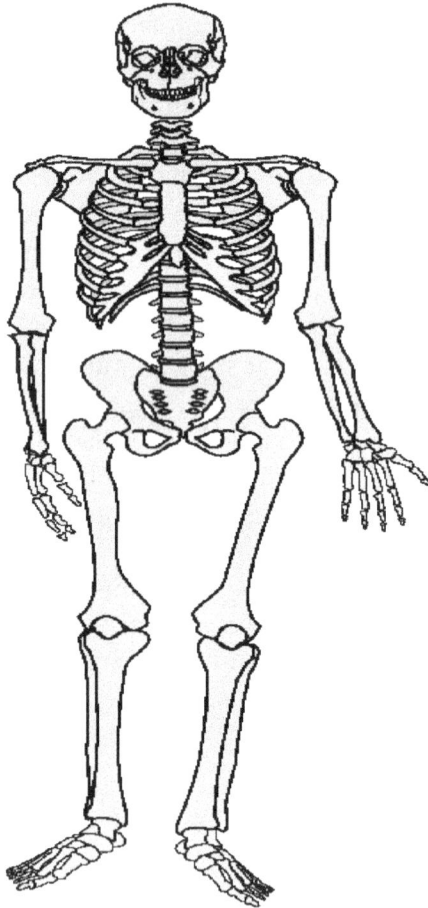

  The skeletal system is the support of the human body. Through this system, hair, skin and nails are all affected. There are 206 bones in the adult human body that store minerals, protect vital organs, and allow movement of the body to occur. Additional parts of the skeleton include cartilage, tendons, ligaments and joints.

  There are four types of bone names according to their shapes: long (humerus), short (wrist), flat (skull) and irregular (vertebrae). A fifth category is sometimes added in certain texts-the sesamoid bone (or round bones like the kneecap.

The joints of the skeletal system are classified according to their structure and type of movement that they provide. Here we have the hinge joint (elbow), the pivot joint (head of radius rotating against ulna), the saddle joint (thumb), the Condyloid joint (C1 and C2 vertebra), the Ball-and-Socket joint (shoulder or hip), and the Gliding joint (processes between the vertebrae).

There are 12 bony landmarks in the human body that protrude from the body that health professionals often use as reference points. These bony landmarks include the Zygomatic bone (cheek bone), the Acromion process of the scapula, the Medial and Lateral epicondyle of the humerus, the iliac crest (top of the hip bone), the Styloid process of the radius and ulna (felt at the wrist), the Patella (kneecap), the Anterior border of the tibia (right underneath the kneecap on the top front of the lower leg), the Lateral malleolus of fibula and the Medial malleolus of tibia (ankle) and the Calcaneus (heel).

Every bone in the human body connects to at least one other bone in one way or the other except for one-the hyoid. The hyoid is anchored by the tongue.

Note all skeletons are created equal. A trained eye can tell the difference between a female skeleton and a male skeleton. These differences include:

1. Size-male skeletons are generally larger than female ones

2. Shape of Pelvis-female skeletons has broader and shallower pelvises while male skeletons have a deep and narrow skeleton.

3. Size of Pelvic Inlet-female skeletons has a wider pelvic inlet than men do so that the baby can pass through it more easily.

4. Pubic angle-female skeletons generally have a wider pubic angle then men do

## Common Pathogens

| Disease/Ailment | Description |
|---|---|
| Arthritis | Inflammation of a joint |
| Bunion | Inflammation of the bursa of the big toe |
| Carpal Tunnel | Compression of the nerve and ligaments of the wrist |
| Fracture | Broken bone |
| Ganglion cyst | Fluid-filled synovial sacks found on joint capsules and tendons |
| Gout | Inflammation of the joints caused by excessive uric acid in the body |
| Myeloma | Malignant tumor of the bone marrow |
| Osteoarthritis | Degeneration of bones and joint due to arthritis |
| Osteporosis | Loss of bone density and thinning of bone tissue |
| Rheumatoid arthritis | Autoimmune disorder with inflammation of joints |
| Spondylosis | Degenerative condition of the vertebrae column |
| Sprain | Damage to the ligaments surrounding a joint due to overstretching |
| Whiplash | Injury to the cervical spine due to violent movement |

Essential oils can help bones that are inflamed or in pain. Essential oils for this system include lavender, chamomile, helichrysum, cypress, juniper and grapefruit

### Essential Oils for Arthritis and Arthritic Pain

| Essential Oil | Function |
| --- | --- |
| Basil | Good for arthritis and rheumatism, muscle spasm and gout. |
| Cedarwood | Decongests the lymph system, unblocks arteries, breaks down fat deposits, and improves poor circulation. Reduces fluid retention. |
| Clove Bud | Analgesic (pain relief). Arthritis and muscle cramps. |
| Eucalyptus | Reduces fluid retention. Eases muscle aches and rheumatism |
| Fennel | Good for lymph and fluid retention. Improves circulation. |
| Frankincense | Relieves muscle aches and pain caused by rheumatism. Helps anxiety, asthma, bronchitis, stress, scars and stretch marks. |
| Geranium | Reduces fluid retention, balances hormones, and eases anxiety, depression and nervous tension. Stimulates circulation. |
| Lavender | Good for headaches, insomnia and inflammation. |
| Lemon | Cleanse and detoxify. Makes the body more alkaline helping arthritis, gout, rheumatism, pain and inflammation of the joints. |
| Lemongrass | Boosts the immune system, tones muscles, relieves tired aching legs and eliminates lactic acid build-up. Tendons, ligaments |
| Palmarosa | Anti-viral and Anti-fungal. Cellular stimulant, relieves stiff and sore muscles, uplifting and stress reducing. |
| Peppermint | Cooling and Pain relieving. Good for headaches and pain in general. Great for muscular aches and pains. Inflammation |
| Rosemary | Warming oil aids in stimulating the circulatory system and tones muscles. Rub into joints to ease |

| | |
|---|---|
| | pain. Reduces cellulite, gout pain, fatigue, and fluid retention. |
| Tea Tree | Anti-bacterial, Anti-fungal, Painful joints, muscle aches. |
| Helichrysum | Inflammation, muscle cramps, arthritis |
| Pepper | Inflammation |
| Hyssop | Inflammation |
| Windtergreen | Reduce pain of arthritis and muscle cramps |

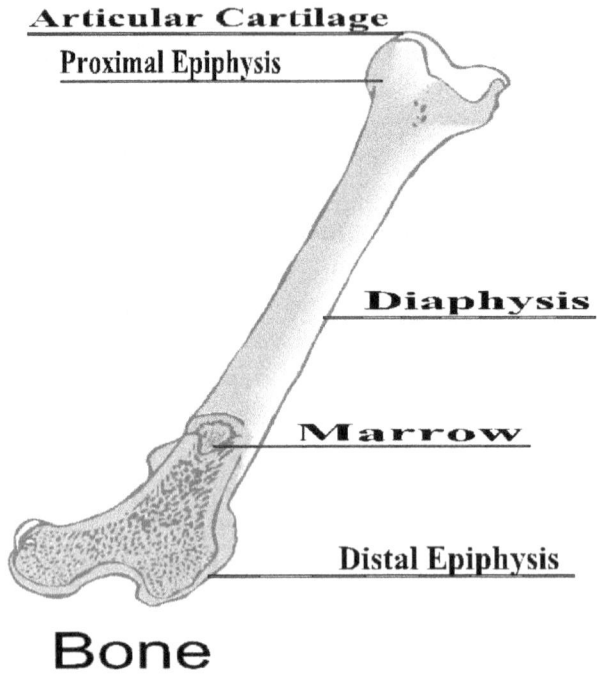

**Articular Cartilage**

Proximal Epiphysis

**Diaphysis**

**Marrow**

Distal Epiphysis

Bone

**The Immune System**

The main responsibility of the Immune System is to identify foreign invaders and neutralize them. The immune system includes the digestive system, integumentary system, cardiovascular system, endocrine system and the lymphatic system. The cells of the immune system are called *lymphocytes.* Lymphocytes are broken down into two major cells-the B cells and T-cells and are manufactured in the bone marrow. The T-cells, and a subgroup called *killer cells*, are created to fight invading pathogens. Pathogens include everything from viruses and bacteria to parasitic worms and cancer.

Disorders of the immune system include autoimmune diseases (Hashimoto's thyroiditis), inflammatory diseases (rheumatoid arthritis), and immunodeficiency (HIV/AIDS). Addition ailments include diabetes, and lupus.

Essential oils can help boost the immunity system by reducing stress levels and calming the nervous system. Oils can also help with autoimmune disease, allergies, hives, rashes, chronic fatigue and viral illnesses. Essential oils can help boost the immunity system by reducing stress levels and calming the nervous system. Oils can also help with autoimmune disease, allergies, hives, rashes, chronic fatigue and viral illnesses.

In the immune system, aromatherapy can be used in two ways. One way is to oppose the threatening pathogens by using essential oils that are antiviral or antibacterial. Another way to use essential oils is to increase the activity and strengthen the organ and cells that are under attack.

Antibacterial-cinnamon bark, clove, basil, oregano, tea tree, thyme

Antiviral-cinnamon bark, marjoram, tea tree, lavender, peppermint, eucalyptus, sandalwood, lemongrass

Antifungal-lemongrass, Melissa, eucalyptus, geranium, clove, patchouli, petitgrain, spearmint

Depressed Immunity-bay laurel, frankincense, marjoram, lemon, palmarosa, lemongrass, geranium, patchouli

Chronic Fatigue-Black spruce, pine, ginger, rosemary, cardamom, frankincense

Allergies-chamomile, cedar, turmeric, lavender, tea tree

Candidiasis-geranium, patchouli, palmarosa
Viral Infections-eucalyptus, marjoram, tea tree, ravensara,
ginger, cardamon

Use the following essential oils to build up the strength of the following organs:

Spleen-black pepper, lavender
Adrenal Gland-rosemary, geranium

**NOTE:** If you have depleted your immune system it may take you at least one month of use before you start to feel better. It does take time to strengthen a weakened immune system because there are so many systems involved in the process and you must consider these other systems when deciding on what oils to use and how to use them.

# Common Pathogens

| Disease/Ailment | Description |
| --- | --- |
| Adhesion | Built up of layers of fascial tissue |
| Atrophy | Loss of muscle mass/strength due to immobility |
| Bursitis | Inflammation of a bursa |
| Contracture | Shortening of muscle fibers, tendons or fascia |
| Cramps | Involuntary and painful muscle twitch (spasm) |
| Fibromyalgia | Chronic condition of pain and aching muscles-18 points |
| Hernia | Tear in muscle wall that allows an organ to protrude |
| Muscular Dystrophy (MS) | Chronic, genetic diseases causing muscles to degenerate and weaken ending in atrophy |
| Myasthenia gravis | Autoimmune muscle disease causing weakness/fatigue |
| Repetitive Motion Disorder | Damage to joints, muscles, etc. due to repetitive motions. |
| Scar Tissue | Collagen fibers laid down over areas of injury in muscle |
| Spasms | Sudden and violent muscle contraction. A cramp. |
| Sprain | Acute injury to ligaments around joints (whiplash) |
| Strains | Injury or tear in muscle, tendon and attachments to bone |
| Tendinitis | Inflammation of a tendon after repetitive movements |
| Tetanus | Bacterial disease causing locking of the jaw |
| TMJ | Muscle contraction of the jaw |

# The Genita-Urinary System

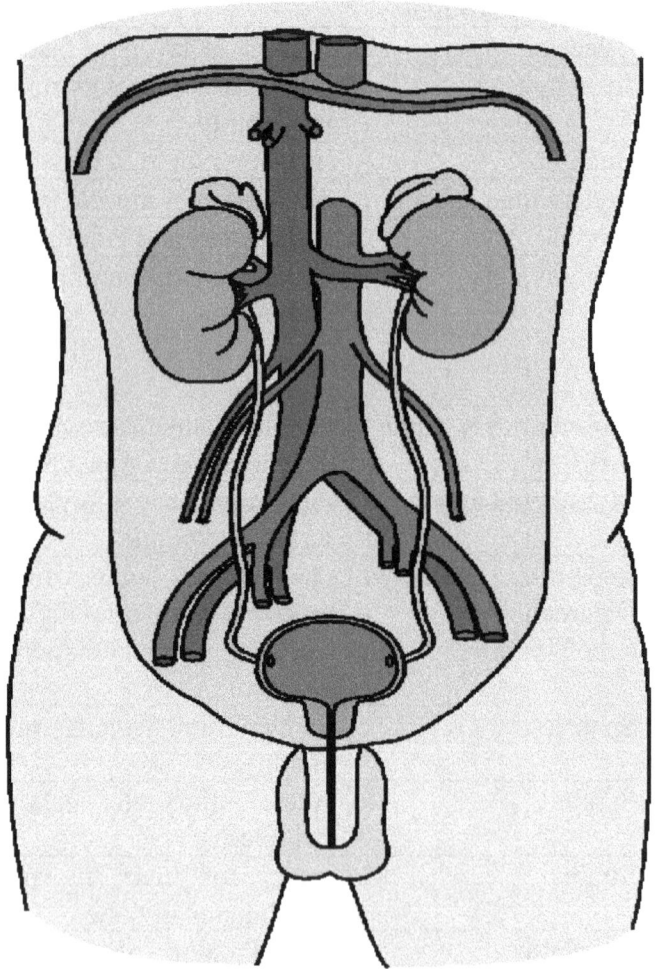

The Urinary System is responsible for making urine, filtering and removing waste products, adjusting water and electrolytes levels and maintaining the correct pH levels in the body.

The organs of the urinary system include the two kidneys, two ureters, one urinary bladder, and one urethra. The bean-shaped kidneys are the primary organs of the urinary system and they perform several functions in the body.

Their first function is to filter the blood of waster products. The second function is to produce urine to carry the waste products out of the body. The third function of the kidneys is to regulate blood pressure and volume by maintaining water balance in the body. And lastly, the kidneys regulate red blood cell production by secreting erythropoietin (EPO).

In the body, the right kidney is usually a little lower than the left. These organs begin to lose functional nephron unite and weight in adult over the age of 35. By age 85, there is approximately a 30% reduction in kidney mass. This decrease in function may make it harder for older people to filter and excrete medications from their blood. So when working with an older individual, adjust medications accordingly.

*Urinalysis* is the physical, chemical and microscopic examination of urine. The urine can tell a lot about what is going in the body. Physical characteristics of urine include color, order, cloudiness, and density. Abnormally dark urine signal excess bile pigments that may come from a diseased liver or internal bleeding. Below are the normal characteristics of urine:

Color-transparent yellow, amber or straw colored
Odor-slight
pH-4.6-8.0
Gravity-1.001-1.035
Compounds-
Mineral ions (Na+, CI-, K+)
Nitrogenous wastes (ammonia, creatinine, urea, uric acid)
Suspended solids (sediments): bacteria, blood cells, casts
Urine pigments

**Terms of the Urinary System:**
Urination or Voiding-passage of urine from the body or the emptying of the bladder.
Enuresis-involuntary urination (bed wetting)
Anuria-absence of urine
Oliguria-scanty amounts of urine
Polyuria-large amount of urine
Renal failure- Kidneys cannot clear blood of urea or waste products. Toxic condition occurs.
Urinary incontinence- Leakage of urine caused by age and weakened sphincter muscles.
Uremia-Terminal stage of renal failure

Essential oils to use for the urinary tract infection include those to help in the elimination of excess fluid in the body, those that stimulate the circulatory and lymphatic systems of the body and those that help with inflammation, irritation and pain. Methods of application include Sitz baths, baths, compresses, and massage oils.

Analgesic-R. chamomile, peppermint, lavender, marjoram
Antimicrobial-Frankincense, bergamot, lemon, thyme linalol
Antibacterial-peppermint, lemongrass, cinnamon bark, thyme CT thymol
Anti-inflammatory-R. chamomile, lavender sandalwood.
Antiviral-eucalyptus, ginger, pine, tea tree, Niaouli, ravensara, black pepper
Antispasmodic-clary sage, petitgrain, marjoram, basil, tarragon, frankincense

Other oils to consider include Cajeput, Eucalyptus, Rosewood, sage and Juniper berries.

Urinary Tract Infection: lavender, geranium, myrrh, sandalwood and tea tree can be used in an abdominal and low-back massage or used in baths.

## Common Pathogens

| Disease/Ailment | Description |
|---|---|
| Cystitis | Inflammation of the bladder due to bacteria |
| Glomerulonephritis | Inflammation of the kidneys |
| Kidney stones | Deposits of calculi (mineral salts) in the kidneys |
| Polycystic kidney | Formation of noncancerous cysts in the kidneys |
| Pyelonephritis | Infection of the kidney and renal pelvis |
| Urinary tract infection (UTI) | Infection of any organ of the urinary system. |

## The Reproductive System

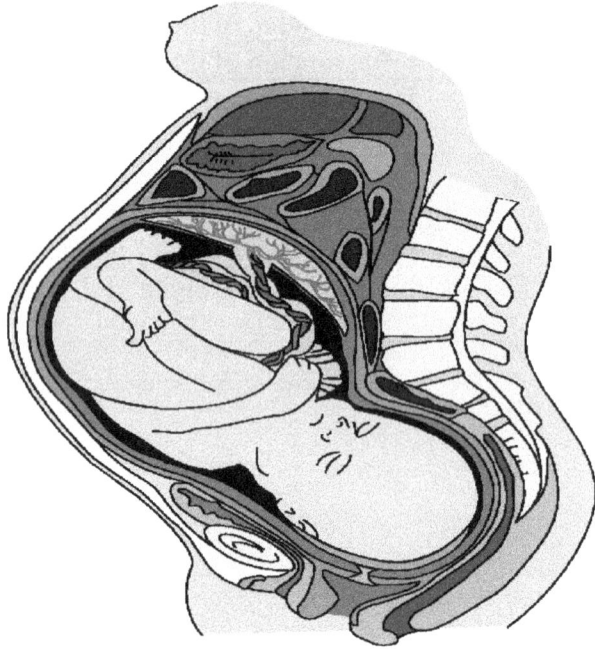

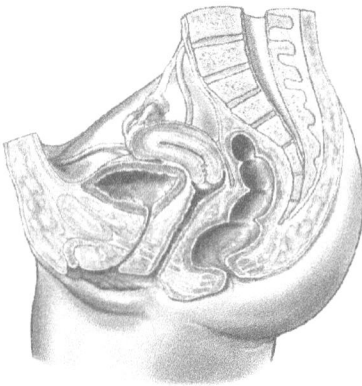

**Female**

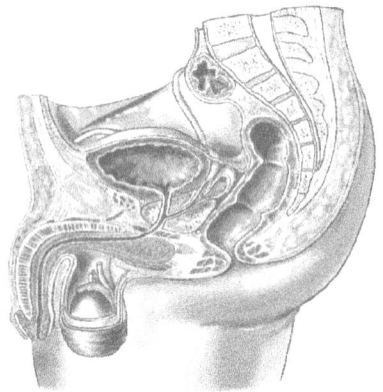

**Male**

The Reproductive System includes the regulation of hormones, ovaries, uterus, and the menstrual cycle, pregnancy and menopause.

This system ensures the survival of the species by protecting the genes that characterize who and what we are as a human being. A potential part of this system is called the Sexual Reproduction system. In Sexual reproduction, two parent organisms (male and female) come together to contribute half of the chromosomes needed to create an offspring. The male contributes the sperm and the female contributes and egg, or ovum. When these two items fuse together in a process called fertilization, they form an offspring cell called a *zygote*.

The essential reproductive organs for men and woman are called *gonads*. For the men, the gonads consist of a pair of main sex glands called the tests which produce spermatozoa. The testes secrete the male hormone testosterone which has masculinizing characteristics.

For women, the essential reproductive organ is the paired ovaries which produce the female sex cell called *ova*. Accessory organs of reproduction in woman consist of mammary glands (breasts), external genitals and a series of ducts that extend from near the ovaries to the exterior. External genitals include the mons pubis, clitoris, external urinary meatus, openings of vestibular glands, orifice of vagina, labia minora and majora, hymen, and the perineum.

The menstrual cycle involves the uterus, ovaries, vagina and breasts. Every 28 days (more or less), the menstrual cycle goes through a variety of changes. When a woman begins her first day of flow, this is day 1 of the menstrual cycle. For days 1-4 of the cycle, called the *menses*, there is a sloughing of bits of endometrium (uterine lining) with bleeding. Following is the *proliferative phase* represents the days between the end of menses and ovulation. Ovulation generally occurs in the middle of the woman's menses around the 15th day (more or less). This is the time of the month where the woman is most fertile and able to conceive. It is the combine action of the anterior pituitary hormone FSH and LH that causing ovulation to occur. The *secretory phase* represents the days between ovulation and beginning of next menses. Here comes a sharp decrease in estrogen and progesterone that brings on menstruation of a pregnancy does not occur.

## Sexually transmitted diseases

Sexually transmitted diseases (STD) are the most common of all communicable diseases and are caused by a variety of organisms. These include AIDS, candidiasis, genital herpes and warts, gonorrhea, hepatitis, scabies, and syphilis, among others.

## Essential oils for this body system:

Essential oils often used to help this body system include antispasmodics for cramping, emmenagogue for menses, anti-inflammatory and vasoconstrictors for endometriosis, and distressing oils for PMS, stress and tensions

Calming-rose, lavender, linden blossom, sandalwood, neroli, cr. hamomile, patchouli, bitter orange

Estrogenic-aniseed, geranium, fennel, sage, lemongrass, Melissa

Anti-spasmodic-basil, cardamom, ginger, black pepper, clove, marjoram, rosemary, clary sage, fennel

Emmonagogues-basil, rosemary, juniper, fennel, peppermint, sage, thyme

Dysmenorrhea-r. chamomile, ginger, black pepper, peppermint

PMS-aniseed, geranium, grapefruit, juniper, black spruce, frankincense, fennel, sage, melissa, sandalwood

Urinary Tract Infection-lavender, geranium, sandalwood, tea tree

Edema-geranium, lemon, cypress, grapefruit

Stretch Marks-lavender, mandarin, helichrysum, neroli

Postnatal Depression-lemon, grapefruit, rose, marjoram, ylang ylang

Leg Cramps-petitgrain, marjoram, black pepper, clary sage, lavender

Morning Sickness-ginger, peppermint

Constipation-ginger, black pepper, sweet orange, rosemary, fennel

Varicose Veins-cypress, geranium, lemon

Common Pathogens

| Disease/Ailment | Description |
|---|---|
| Breast cancer | Malignant tumor of the breast |
| Cervical cancer | Malignant growth in the cervix caused by the human pupilloma virus (HPV). Sexually transmitted virus. |
| Cryptorchidism | Undescended testes |
| Dysmenorrhea | Painful cramping with menses |
| Erectile dysfunction | Failure to achieve erection of the penis |
| Endometrial cancer | Cancer of the endometrial lining of the uterus |
| Fibrocystic breast disease | Benign cysts form in the breasts |
| Fibroid Tumor | Benign fibrous growth occurring in the uterus |
| Hydrocele | Accumulation of watery fluid in the socrum |
| Hypospadias | Urethra opens on underside of glans or shaft |
| Inguinal hernia | Protrusion of abdominopelvic organs |
| Mastitis | Inflammation of the breasts |
| Memorrhagia | Excessive bleeding during menses |
| Ogligospermia | Low sperm production |
| Ovarian cancer | Cancer of the ovary |
| Ovarian cyst | Cyst developing in the ovary |
| Paraphimosis | Foreskin cannot be replaced to usual position after it has been retracted behing the glans |
| Pelvic inflammatory disease (PID) | Inflammation of the female reproductive organs |
| Phimosis | Tight foreskin cannot be retracted over glans |
| Preeclampsia | Toxemia of pregnancy resulting in hypertension, headaches and edema. |
| Premenstrual syndrome (PMS) | Problems that occur 1-2 weeks before menses that include bloating, headaches, edema, depression, etc. |
| Prolapsed uterus | Fallen uterus that may cause the cervix to protrude through the vaginal opening |
| Prostate cancer | Malignancy of the prostate tissue |
| Testicular cancer | Cancer of the testes |

**Chapter Seven**
**Therapeutics**


**Pharmacologic Properties**
Essential oils contain certain properties that make them medicinal in nature. Recent studies have shown great success in using essential oils to prevent the transmission of some staphylococcus, streptococcus and candida.

Some of the medicinal ingredients in plants include menthol, capsaicin, anise and camphor. Essential oils containing these ingredients work on the upper respiratory system of the body and act as mild expectorants, decongestants and antitussives (Capable of relieving or suppressing coughing). Some oils have a diuretic effect (juniper), eugenol effect (clove oil to numb tooth aches), or antiseptic effects (thymol).

**Materia Medica**
*Materia medica* is a Latin term that means a collection of knowledge about the therapeutic properties of substances used for healing. Homeopathy has its own material medica. The term was believed to have been first used in the 1st century AD by the Greek physician Pedanius Dioscorides in his writings, *De material medica* (on medical materials). Today, the words '*material medica*' have been replaced by the word, pharmacology. Pharmacology is the science of drugs (their composition, uses, and effects) as it is concerned with medicine and healing. It is also the study of the preparation, properties, uses and actions of drugs, as well as, their interactions with living organisms.

**Actions**
On the next page is information that I retrieved from www.wikipedia.com on the antimicrobial properties of 21 essential oils and two plant essences. The chart below shows how these oils and plant essences stood up against five food-borne pathogens.

| Pharmacology: major drug groups | |
|---|---|
| Gastrointestinal tract/ metabolism (A) | stomach acid<br>Antacids<br>$H_2$ antagonists<br>Proton pump inhibitors<br>Antiemetics, Laxatives<br>Antidiarrhoeals/Antipropulsives<br>Anti-obesity drugs<br>Anti-diabetics<br>Vitamins and Dietary minerals |
| Blood and blood forming organs (B) | Antithrombotics<br>Antiplatelets<br>Anticoagulants<br>Thrombolytics/fibrinolytics<br>Antihemorrhagics<br>Platelets<br>Coagulants<br>Antifibrinolytics |
| Cardiovascular system (C) | *cardiac therapy/antianginals*<br>Cardiac glycosides<br>Antiarrhythmics<br>Cardiac stimulants<br>Antihypertensives<br>Diuretics<br>Vasodilators<br>Beta blockers<br>Calcium channel blockers<br>*renin-angiotensin system*<br>ACE inhibitors<br>Angiotensin II receptor antagonists<br>Renin inhibitors<br>Antihyperlipidemics<br>Statins<br>Fibrates<br>Bile acid sequestrants |
| Skin (D) | Emollients<br>Cicatrizants |

| | |
|---|---|
| | Antipruritics<br>Antipsoriatics<br>Medicated dressings |
| Genitourinary system (G) | Hormonal contraception<br>Fertility agents<br>SERMs<br>Sex hormones |
| Endocrine system (H) | Hypothalamic-pituitary hormones<br>Corticosteroids<br>Glucocorticoids<br>Mineralocorticoids<br>Sex hormones<br>Thyroid hormones/Antithyroid agents |
| Infections and infestations (J, P, QI) | Antimicrobials: Antibacterials (Antimycobacterials)<br>Antifungals, Antivirals<br>Antiparasitics<br>Antiprotozoals<br>Anthelmintics<br>Ectoparasiticides<br>IVIG<br>Vaccines |
| Malignant disease (L01-L02) | Anticancer agents<br>Antimetabolites<br>Alkylating<br>Spindle poisons<br>Antineoplastic<br>Topoisomerase inhibitors |
| Immune disease (L03-L04) | Immunomodulators<br>Immunostimulants<br>Immunosuppressants |
| Muscles, bones, and joints (M) | Anabolic steroids<br>Anti-inflammatories , NSAIDs<br>Antirheumatics<br>Corticosteroids<br>Muscle relaxants<br>Bisphosphonates |

| Brain and nervous system (N) | Analgesics |
| --- | --- |
| | Anesthetics, General, Local |
| | Anorectics |
| | Anti-ADHD Agents |
| | Antiaddictives |
| | Anticonvulsants |
| | Antidementia Agents |
| | Antidepressants |
| | Antimigraine Agents |
| | Antiparkinson's Agents |
| | Antipsychotics |
| | Anxiolytics |
| | Depressants |
| | Entactogens, Entheogens |
| | Euphoriants |
| | Hallucinogens, Psychedelics |
| | Dissociatives |
| | Deliriants |
| | Hypnotics/Sedatives |
| | Mood Stabilizers |
| | Neuroprotectives |
| | Nootropics |
| | Neurotoxins |
| | Orexigenics |
| | Serenics |
| | Stimulants |
| | Wakefulness-Promoting Agents |
| Respiratory system (R) | Decongestants |
| | Bronchodilators |
| | Cough medicines |
| | $H_1$ antagonists |
| Sensory organs (S) | Ophthalmologicals |
| | Otologicals |
| Other ATC (V) | Antidotes |
| | Contrast media |
| | Radiopharmaceuticals |
| | Dressings |

**Chapter Eight**
**Safety**

Because essential oils have pharmacological benefits to them, they should be used and handled with care. Some essential oils are applied directly to the skin, some are inhaled and others are used on pets, or for cooking. Some oils can cause allergic reactions when applied to skin of both humans and animals, so these should be used with care. Oils that can cause allergic reaction over time are called photosensitive, photosensitizers, or skin sensitive. Oils that may prove harmful over long usage, and in fact, may result in a toxic build-up in the liver, is called hepatoxic.

Essential oils (outside of Lavender and Tea Tree) should ever be applied directly from the bottle to the skin. This is called Neat. Before applying essential oils to the skin, they should be mixed with carrier oils such as olive oil, sweet almond oil, etc. We will cover some basic dilution ratios in the chapters to come.

Great care should be taken when giving essential oils to women who are pregnant or nursing, children, pets, people with high or low blood pressure and those who are epileptic or suffer from seizures. Please refer to the list of contraindication before giving certain essentials to your family or clients.

**Handling**

Since essential oils can be hazardous to specific groups of people, I am sure to wear gloves when I work with them. Since essential oils can be absorbed by the skin, I am sure to be cautious about what essentials, and how much of it, that I allow to be absorbed into my skin. This is especially important to massage therapists who use essential oils in their lotions and creams and massage several clients in one day, day after day. Therapists are absorbing these substances into their body on a daily basis. Wouldn't it be advantageous for them to know what risks they are also taking on?

It is also important to use glass containers and syringes when working with essential oils. Avoid rubbers and plastics as some oils can degrade those materials. The best equipment to use is a chemistry syringe that has a seal and piston that wipes off the essential oil from the wall of the pipette. These syringes are more accurate in measuring the amount of oils that you are actually using and because of that, facilitate better quality control.

**Skin Testing-The Patch Test**
You should never use essential oils directly on your skin, they should be diluted first. One way to test your blend on yourself, or the person who you are making a blend for, is called a **Patch Test**. To perform the Patch Test, you will apply a drop of the oil (mixed with a carrier oil that you created), on the inside of the forearm.

Cover the drop with a simple bandage and wait 24 hours. After the 24 hour waiting period, remove the bandage and see if there was any reaction on the skin. If there was no reaction, this means that you (or your client) is most likely not sensitive to the oil, or blend that you have created.

**Note:**
Some of the best places to use the Patch Test are on the most sensitive areas of your body which include the inside of the elbow, back of the wrist, or under the arm. If you do suffer from a reaction, wash with the area with soap and water.

**Standard Precautions**
- General Do's and Don'ts
- Do not take essential oils internally
- Keep essential oils out of the reach of children and pets
- Keep essential oils out of your eyes and mucous membranes
- Always dilute essential oils in a carrier oil (never apply oils directly to your skin)
- Be sure to use 100% pure essential oils.
- People with Epilepsy should avoid such essential oils as rosemary, and sage.
- If you are taking Staten medications-avoid hepatoxic oils such as grapefruit.
- Remember that citrus oils are photosensitive. Stay out of sunlight for 4-5 hours after applying essential oils. Also, avoid tanning beds when using citrus oils.
- People with estrogenic cancers should avoid such essential oils as rose, clary sage and geranium.
- People with high blood pressure, or those who are taking blood thinner, should avoid the oils of cinnamon, sage and hyssop.
- Asthma sufferers should avoid steam inhalation as this may irritate and aggravate the mucus membranes. Avoid essential oil of thyme.
- Avoid prolonged use of essential oils. Have 5-6 days on and take 1-2 days off.
- Avoid the essential oil of pine if you have prostate concerns.
- Store essential oils in colored glass containers out of direct sunlight.
- Be sure to use proper dosages for children and pets-do not use adult dosages.
- Be sure to have proper ventilation when using essential oils over a long period of time.
- Be sure to perform a Patch Test on yourself before applying essential oils to your entire body, especially if you have sensitive skin.
- Always check with your client about their past reactions to using essential oils.

- Refrigerate carrier oils to prevent them from becoming rancid.
- Old oils are more prone to cause skin reactions. Throw these oils out. Some oils like patchouli and sandalwood get better with age- most do not.
- If you keep a bird in your home, stay away from using essential oils in a diffuser.
- Use caution during pregnancy and while nursing. Safe essential oils include lavender, mandarin and Roman Chamomile.

## Emergency Issues

### What to do for reactions:

If you accidentally ingest an essential oil, call your local Poison Control Center. Do NOT induce vomiting or give liquids to drink.

If a skin reaction or irritation appears, stop using essential oils. Some essential oils like cinnamon, oregano, fennel, clove and verbena can cause skin irritation. The best relief from skin irritations due to essential oils is to apply a fatty oil, such as coconut, which will dilute the essential oil.

If you accidentally get an essential oil in your eye-don't rub it! Instead, soak a cotton ball into milk or vegetable oil and place it in the affected area. You can also try to use coconut oil, olive oil, cooking oil or milk. Wipe outward from the eye. You can also choose to flush the eye area with lukewarm water for 15 minutes. If pain persists, seek medical advice immediately.

Avoid overexposure to essential oils by being sure there is proper ventilation. Should you feel dizzy or nauseous, get some fresh air.

Some oils on photosensitive (such as the citrus oils). Avoid sunlight and tanning beds 3-4 hours after applying these oils to your body. Should sunburn occur, apply aloe vera gel gently and sparingly to the area and avoid any addition heat to the area.

Before using a new essential oil-read all about it. Read about its properties, dosages and contraindications. Then decide if it is right for you.

**What if I spill essential oils on my furniture?**

You must take care when using essential oils around furniture as some oils will remove the finish. Should essential oils spill on your furniture, quickly remove it with a tissue or paper towel.

**Overdose**

It never ceases to amaze me that the same people who believe that essential oils have healing properties to them, don't believe that they can over dose on them. You have to first remember that essential oils are 50-70 times more concentrated than herbs. It is also important to remember that while some essential oils like Ylang Ylang are sedative in small doses and that is large doses they have the opposite effect and can be simulative.

There are many conflicting reports of injury and death form essential oils but there is little scientific research that has been done on the subject. I will try to include the information that I can find on the inherent dangers of essential oils.

Too much nutmeg can make you hallucinate; oregano and cassia can cause your skin to burn. Too much rosemary essential oil can cause you to vomit, kidney irritation, muscle spasms, bleeding from the uterus, coma and even death. Pennyroyal may cause seizures, liver damage, lung damage, loss of consciousness and even death.

Eucalyptus oil can cause a burning sensation in your mouth, difficulty swallowing, seizure, drowsiness, skin irritant; can induce labor in pregnant women, shallow or rapid breathing, weak heartbeat, and swelling.

Bergamot oil can cause blurred vision, burning sensation, muscle cramping, tingling sensations and even paresthesia (altered sensations). Other essential oils that can be potentially lethal when consumed in great amounts include arnica, bitter almond, birch, camphor, mustard, parsley, peppermint, tansy, turmeric, wintergreen and wormseed.

In case of overdose, call for emergency medical assistance (911). Do not induce vomiting unless instructed by medical professional. Be sure to keep the bottle, or bottles of oils that the person has overdosed on so that you can give them to the attending medical professional.

Depending on the person and the essential oil that they have overdosed on, the person should see improvement after treatment to within days of the overdose.

**Preventing Essential Oil Overdose**

There are many things that you can do to prevent accidently overdosing on essential oils. Some of the same things that you can do to prevent overdosing on essential oils is the same things that you would do to prevent overdosing on other drugs.

- Follow the instructions on the bottle and your therapist.
- Always take the proper dosage.

### Individual Oil and their Precaution

| Essential Oil | Precautions |
| --- | --- |
| Basil | Avoid during pregnancy, epilepsy, photosensitive |
| Cassia | Photosensitive, irritates nasal membranes |
| Citrus Oils | Photosensitive |
| Clove | Photosensitive, avoid during pregnancy |
| Clary Sage | Avoid during pregnancy |
| Coriander | May cause nausea |
| Eucalyptus | Avoid during pregnancy or nursing |
| Fennel | Avoid during pregnancy, seizures |
| Ginger | Skin sensitizing |
| Grapefruit | Photosensitive |
| Lemongrass | Skin sensitizing |
| Marjoram | Diminishes sex drive and function, drowsiness |
| Melissa | Skin sensitizing |
| Oregano | Skin sensitizing, avoid during pregnancy |
| Peppermint | Avoid with high blood pressure and homeopathy |
| Roman Chamomile | Avoid during pregnancy |
| Rosemary | Avoid during pregnancy, high blood pressure, epilepsy |
| Tansy | Allergic Reactions |
| Thyme | Avoid during pregnancy, high blood pressure. Skin sensitizing |
| Wintergreen | Avoid during pregnancy, epilepsy |

**Chapter Nine**
**Delivery Methods**

**Application of Essential Oils**
Please remember that essential oils remain in the body for 20-90 minutes. Essential oils are naturally excreted from the body through exhalation, urine, and sweat. Below is a list of common uses for essential oils:

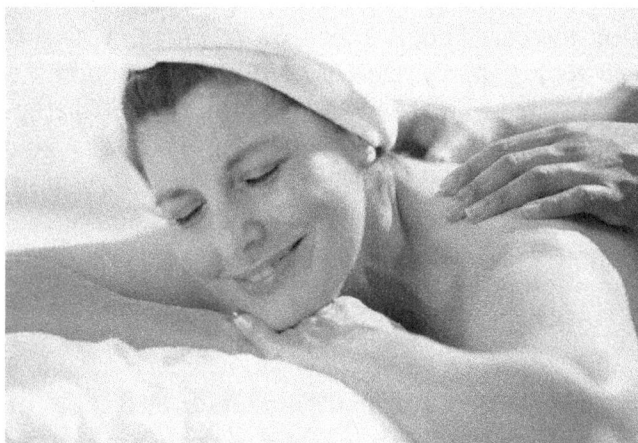

Add essential oils in a carrier oil, cream or lotion for a massage session

**Topical Use:** applying essential oils to the skin of the body.
Since the skin is the largest organ of the body, applying essential oil to the skin just makes sense. The skin is able to rapidly absorb the essential oil and bring it into the bloodstream. This is possible because essential oils are lipotropic (fat soluble). Also, you can massage the essential oil in a blend directly on an area of need such as massaging the abdomen for digestive problems, or massaging an area of a sore muscle, an injury, the temples for a headache, etc.

Benefits of massage include:
- Enters the blood stream within 3 minutes.
- Apply to a specific area (muscle leg cramp) or to the entire body.

- Increases lymph system
- Increases circulation system
- Prolonged use may cause phototoxicity or cause skin irritations.

**Massage oil or lotions**-Add essential oils to your massage oils, lotions or creams, and massage into the client, or onto affected area. Aside from massaging the area in need directly, massaging the feet will also help the client as all of the organs and organ tissues are located on the bottoms of the feet, the palms of the hand and on point on the ear. This is called *Reflexology*. You client may also be able to just apply the oil blend to the bottoms of their feet before bedtime. This will also work when a therapist is doing Acupressure. Just add 1-3 drops of oil blend to your finger (or thumb) and press and activate the acupressure point. One last thing that you can do in the massage session with your oils is called *layering*. In layering, you may use one oil blend on the body first, and then when that oil blend dries, you will be able to use another oil blend over top of it. This works especially well on sore muscles where you can use rosemary to calm the muscle spasm and then peppermint to invigorate, etc.

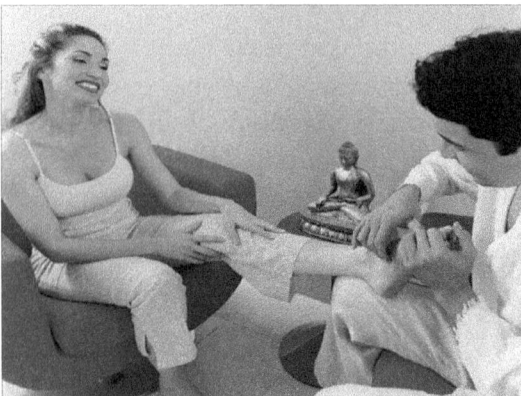

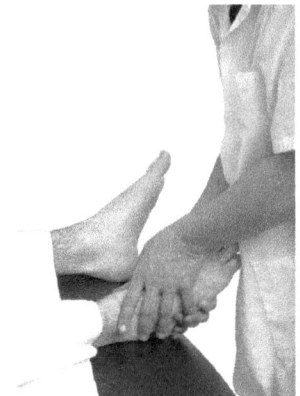

**Reflexology and Foot Massages are great ways to apply oil blends**

**Salves-**Using Golden Salve, Rescue Remedy Creams, etc., you can add essential oils to the salve to use on specific areas of the body in need.

**Compresses (hot and cold)-**You can a few drops of essential oil to a bowl of hot (or cold) water, soak a towel in it, wring it out, and place the towel on the area in need. A simple fever reducing recipe would be to use 4oz. of cold water, 2 drops of lemon, 1 drop of peppermint and 1 drop of lavender essential oil. Dip washcloth or towel into the water, wring it out and apply to the forehead, neck, under the armpits, or the bottoms of the feet. Leave on until towel warms (usually 5-10 minutes) and repeat.

**Bath-**to use essential oils in the bath, you must add the essential oil to a carrier such as bath salts, Epsom salts, carrier oils, or vodka. Be sure to remember that you while you can safely use essential oils in the bathtub for adults, great care must be taken in what oils you use for children and babies and how much is considered safe. Some oils can be toxic for children and pets so please do not use these oils. See list of precautions listed earlier in this manual.

Baths are excellent for skin problems, circulation problems, respiratory problems, stress and nervous tension, muscle aches and pains, PMS, insomnia, and more. Mix essential oils in with Epson salts or sea salts before adding to the bath (normally 5-12 drops of essential oil per bath). Prolonged use of essential oils may cause irritation.

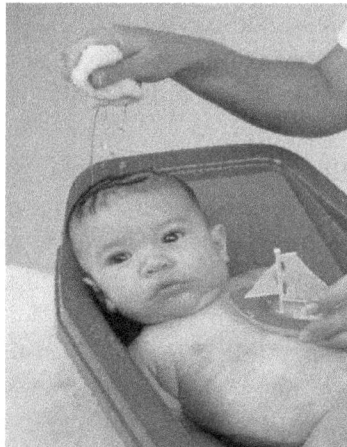

**Baths**-Use less essential oil in baths for children and pets

**Foot Baths**-Add essential oils of lavender and tea tree to a small tub of water to fight fungal infections such as athlete's feet.

**Sitz Baths**-Add essential oils to a small tub and sit for hemorrhoid relief.

**Mouthwash**-Dilute essential oil in a glass of water and vodka. Use for mouth infections, cold sores, and bad breath.

**Suppository**-Mix essential oils with a carrier such as Golden Salve and apply to the area. Use to help with colitis, Crohn's disease and yeast infections. Add 1-2 drops of essential oil blend to a gel capsule and insert into body cavity. Use for relief of hemorrhoids and yeast infections.

**Douche**-Prolonged use may cause colonic problems.

**Inhalation:** sniffing the essential directly from the bottle

Through inhalation we can relax or stimulate the nervous system of the body because the aromas that we breathe in affect our brains through the olfactory receptors. The receptors send impulses along olfactory nerves towards the brain where they will be interpreted and acted upon.

The sense of smell is the easiest and quickest ways to active and stimulates the limbic system of the body. Essential oil molecules enter the brain and blood via cranial nerves, nasal membranes and the alveoli in the lungs. This method is best used for respiratory issues, sinus issues and headaches. Prolonged use of concentrated oils may irritate mucus membranes and cause headaches, dizziness, and nausea.

**Cotton ball, potpourri, pine cones, sachets-**Just a drop or two of essential oil to items like a cotton ball and place in drawers and closets.

**Room diffuser or nebulizer**-Perfect for diffusing essential oils into rooms of your home or office. Also can use for the car.

**Room spray, carpet deodorizer**-Always a good one for when the family is sick, or to bring about a certain mood during the holidays. Covers a large area in a very quick time.

Steam (like putting a few drops of essential oils in a pot of very hot water and then placing a towel of your head and over the pot to inhale the steam.

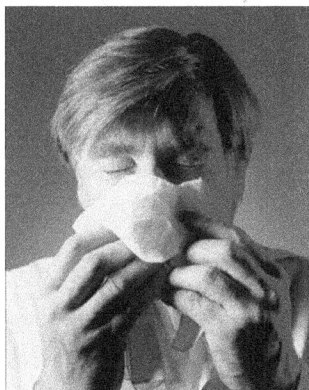

**Inhalation-Inhaling essential oil that was applied to a tissue**

## Oral Ingestion

Because I adhere to the dictates of the National Association of Holistic Aromatherapy (NAHA), I will not give essential oils to people for oral ingestion. But that doesn't mean that all essential oils are unsafe for oral ingestion. I have included a 2013 list of food supplements and additives that the FDA feels are safe for human consumption. The FDA however, has not determined what about of consumption of any one given product is safe. This is why it is important to be under the care of a medical professional should you wish to take essential oils orally. You must also remember that unlike herbs, essential oils are highly concentrated. Most adults dosages range from 1-3 drops no more than 2-3 times a day for up to 5 days and then the body should receive a 'break' from using essential oils.

Essential oils are not recommended for ingestion by people who are pregnant, nursing, children, pets, and epileptics. Oils should be diluted before ingestion in any liquid such as water, tea, or orange juice, but not in milk as milk may make the ingredients inactive.

Some essential oils may burn the membranes of your mouth and esophagus if they are not properly diluted such as cassia, eucalyptus, oregano, ginger and cinnamon. Ingestion of oils is only for a very short period of time and prolonged use may case organ toxicity or damage.

The United States Federal Food, Drug and Cosmetic Act (the Act) has created a sheet called 'Generally Recognized as Safe (GRAS)' that includes substances that are added to food that has received approval by the FDA. The Code of Federal Regulations (CFR) is a codification of the rules of the Food and Drug Administration under Title 21. Under 21 CFR 170.30, food falls under general recognition of food safety through experience and scientific procedures. The CFR at GPO, both current and historical, can also be searched directly at: http://www.gpoaccess.gov/cfr/index.html.

The following information has been taken from the official FDA government Website and lists those essential oils, oleoresins (solvent-free), and natural extractive (including distillates) that are generally recognized as safe for their intended use at: http://www.accessdata.fda.gov/scripts/cdrh/cfdocs/cfcfr/CFRSearch.cfm?fr=182.20

**Note:** Where you see the 'Do' listed below, it means 'ditto.'

| [Code of Federal Regulations] |
|---|
| [Title 21, Volume 3] |
| [Revised as of April 1, 2013] |
| [CITE: 21CFR182.20] |

TITLE 21--FOOD AND DRUGS
CHAPTER I--FOOD AND DRUG ADMINISTRATION
DEPARTMENT OF HEALTH AND HUMAN SERVICES
SUBCHAPTER B--FOOD FOR HUMAN CONSUMPTION (CONTINUED)
PART 182 -- SUBSTANCES GENERALLY RECOGNIZED AS SAFE
Subpart A--General Provisions

Sec. 182.20 Essential oils, oleoresins (solvent-free), and natural extractives (including distillates).

| Essential oils, oleoresins (solvent-free), and natural extractives (including distillates) that are generally recognized as safe for their intended use, within the meaning of section 409 of the Act, are as follows: | |
|---|---|
| Common name | Botanical name of plant source |
| Alfalfa | Medicago sativa L. |

| | |
|---|---|
| Allspice | Pimenta officinalis Lindl. |
| Almond, bitter (free from prussic acid) | Prunus amygdalus Batsch, Prunus armeniaca L., or Prunus persica (L.) Batsch. |
| Ambrette (seed) | Hibiscus moschatus Moench. |
| Angelica root | Angelica archangelica L. |
| Angelica seed and stem | Do. |
| Angostura (cusparia bark) | Galipea officinalis Hancock. |
| Anise | Pimpinella anisum L. |
| Asafetida | Ferula assa-foetida L. and related spp. of Ferula. |
| Balm (lemon balm) | Melissa officinalis L. |
| Balsam of Peru | Myroxylon pereirae Klotzsch. |
| Basil | Ocimum basilicum L. |
| Bay leaves | Laurus nobilis L. |
| Bay (myrcia oil) | Pimenta racemosa (Mill.) J. W. Moore. |
| Bergamot (bergamot orange) | Citrus aurantium L. subsp. bergamia Wright et Arn. |
| Bitter almond (free from prussic acid) | Prunus amygdalus Batsch, Prunus armeniaca L., or Prunus persica (L.) Batsch. |
| Bois de rose | Aniba rosaeodora Ducke. |
| Cacao | Theobroma cacao L. |
| Camomile (chamomile) flowers, Hungarian | Matricaria chamomilla L. |
| Camomile (chamomile) flowers, Roman or English | Anthemis nobilis L. |
| Cananga | Cananga odorata Hook. f. and Thoms. |
| Capsicum | Capsicum frutescens L. and Capsicum annuum L. |
| Caraway | Carum carvi L. |
| Cardamom seed (cardamon) | Elettaria cardamomum Maton. |
| Carob bean | Ceratonia siliqua L. |
| Carrot | Daucus carota L. |
| Cascarilla bark | Croton eluteria Benn. |
| Cassia bark, Chinese | Cinnamomum cassia Blume. |

| | |
|---|---|
| Cassia bark, Padang or Batavia | Cinnamomum burmanni Blume. |
| Cassia bark, Saigon | Cinnamomum loureirii Nees. |
| Celery seed | Apium graveolens L. |
| Cherry, wild, bark | Prunus serotina Ehrh. |
| Chervil | Anthriscus cerefolium (L.) Hoffm. |
| Chicory | Cichorium intybus L. |
| Cinnamon bark, Ceylon | Cinnamomum zeylanicum Nees. |
| Cinnamon bark, Chinese | Cinnamomum cassia Blume. |
| Cinnamon bark, Saigon | Cinnamomum loureirii Nees. |
| Cinnamon leaf, Ceylon | Cinnamomum zeylanicum Nees. |
| Cinnamon leaf, Chinese | Cinnamomum cassia Blume. |
| Cinnamon leaf, Saigon | Cinnamomum loureirii Nees. |
| Citronella | Cymbopogon nardus Rendle. |
| Citrus peels | Citrus spp. |
| Clary (clary sage) | Salvia sclarea L. |
| Clover | Trifolium spp. |
| Coca (decocainized) | Erythroxylum coca Lam. and other spp. of Erythroxylum. |
| Coffee | Coffea spp. |
| Cola nut | Cola acuminata Schott and Endl., and other spp. of Cola. |
| Coriander | Coriandrum sativum L. |
| Cumin (cummin) | Cuminum cyminum L. |
| Curacao orange peel (orange, bitter peel) | Citrus aurantium L. |
| Cusparia bark | Galipea officinalis Hancock. |
| Dandelion | Taraxacum officinale Weber and T. laevigatum DC. |
| Dandelion root | Do. |
| Dog grass (quackgrass, triticum) | Agropyron repens (L.) Beauv. |
| Elder flowers | Sambucus canadensis L. and S. nigra I. |
| Estragole (esdragol, esdragon, tarragon) | Artemisia dracunculus L. |

| | |
|---|---|
| Estragon (tarragon) | Do. |
| Fennel, sweet | Foeniculum vulgare Mill. |
| Fenugreek | Trigonella foenum-graecum L. |
| Galanga (galangal) | Alpinia officinarum Hance. |
| Geranium | Pelargonium spp. |
| Geranium, East Indian | Cymbopogon martini Stapf. |
| Geranium, rose | Pelargonium graveolens L'Her. |
| Ginger | Zingiber officinale Rosc. |
| Grapefruit | Citrus paradisi Macf. |
| Guava | Psidium spp. |
| Hickory bark | Carya spp. |
| Horehound (hoarhound) | Marrubium vulgare L. |
| Hops | Humulus lupulus L. |
| Horsemint | Monarda punctata L. |
| Hyssop | Hyssopus officinalis L. |
| Immortelle | Helichrysum augustifolium DC. |
| Jasmine | Jasminum officinale L. and other spp. of Jasminum. |
| Juniper (berries) | Juniperus communis L. |
| Kola nut | Cola acuminata Schott and Endl., and other spp. of Cola. |
| Laurel berries | Laurus nobilis L. |
| Laurel leaves | Laurus spp. |
| Lavender | Lavandula officinalis Chaix. |
| Lavender, spike | Lavandula latifolia Vill. |
| Lavandin | Hybrids between Lavandula officinalis Chaix and Lavandula latifolin Vill. |
| Lemon | Citrus limon (L.) Burm. f. |
| Lemon balm (see balm) | |
| Lemon grass | Cymbopogon citratus DC. and Cymbopogon lexuosus Stapf. |
| Lemon peel | Citrus limon (L.) Burm. f. |
| Lime | Citrus aurantifolia Swingle. |
| Linden flowers | Tilia spp. |

| | |
|---|---|
| Locust bean | Ceratonia siliqua L, |
| Lupulin | Humulus lupulus L. |
| Mace | Myristica fragrans Houtt. |
| Mandarin | Citrus reticulata Blanco. |
| Marjoram, sweet | Majorana hortensis Moench. |
| Mate | Ilex paraguariensis St. Hil. |
| Melissa (see balm) | |
| Menthol | Mentha spp. |
| Menthyl acetate | Do. |
| Molasses (extract) | Saccarum officinarum L. |
| Mustard | Brassica spp. |
| Naringin | Citrus paradisi Macf. |
| Neroli, bigarade | Citrus aurantium L. |
| Nutmeg | Myristica fragrans Houtt. |
| Onion | Allium cepa L. |
| Orange, bitter, flowers | Citrus aurantium L. |
| Orange, bitter, peel | Do. |
| Orange leaf | Citrus sinensis (L.) Osbeck. |
| Orange, sweet, flowers, peel | Do. |
| Origanum | Origanum spp. |
| Palmarosa | Cymbopogon martini Stapf. |
| Paprika | Capsicum annuum L. |
| Parsley | Petroselinum crispum (Mill.) Mansf. |
| Pepper, black | Piper nigrum L. |
| Pepper, white | Do. |
| Peppermint | Mentha piperita L. |
| Peruvian balsam | Myroxylon pereirae Klotzsch. |
| Petitgrain | Citrus aurantium L. |
| Petitgrain lemon | Citrus limon (L.) Burm. f. |
| Petitgrain mandarin or tangerine | Citrus reticulata Blanco. |
| Pimenta | Pimenta officinalis Lindl. |
| Pimenta leaf | Pimenta officinalis Lindl. |
| Pipsissewa leaves | Chimaphila umbellata Nutt. |

| | |
|---|---|
| Pomegranate | Punica granatum L. |
| Prickly ash bark | Xanthoxylum (or Zanthoxylum) Americanum Mill. or Xanthoxylum clava-herculis L. |
| Rose absolute | Rosa alba L., Rosa centifolia L., Rosa damascena Mill., Rosa gallica L., and vars. of these spp. |
| Rose (otto of roses, attar of roses) | Do. |
| Rose buds and flowers | Do. |
| Rose fruit (hips) | Do. |
| Rose geranium | Pelargonium graveolens L'Her. |
| Rose leaves | Rosa spp. |
| Rosemary | Rosmarinus officinalis L. |
| Saffron | Crocus sativus L. |
| Sage | Salvia officinalis L. |
| Sage, Greek | Salvia triloba L. |
| Sage, Spanish | Salvia lavandulaefolia Vahl. |
| St. John's bread | Ceratonia siliqua L. |
| Savory, summer | Satureia hortensis L. |
| Savory, winter | Satureia montana L. |
| Sloe berries (blackthorn berries) | Prunus spinosa L. |
| Spearmint | Mentha spicata L. |
| Spike lavender | Lavandula latifolia Vill. |
| Tamarind | Tamarindus indica L. |
| Tangerine | Citrus reticulata Blanco. |
| Tarragon | Artemisia dracunculus L. |
| Tea | Thea sinensis L. |
| Thyme | Thymus vulgaris L. and Thymus zygis var. gracilis Boiss. |
| Thyme, white | Do. |
| Thyme, wild or creeping | Thymus serpyllum L. |
| Tuberose | Polianthes tuberosa L. |
| Turmeric | Curcuma longa L. |

| | |
|---|---|
| Vanilla | Vanilla planifolia Andr. or Vanilla tahitensis J. W. Moore. |
| Violet flowers | Viola odorata L. |
| Violet leaves, leaves absolute | Do. |
| Wild cherry bark | Prunus serotina Ehrh. |
| Ylang-ylang | Cananga odorata Hook. f. and Thoms. |

[42 FR 14640, Mar. 15, 1977, as amended at 44 FR 3963, Jan. 19, 1979; 47 FR 29953, July 9, 1982; 48 FR 51613, Nov. 10, 1983; 50 FR 21043 and 21044, May 22, 1985]

**Chapter Ten**
**Blending**

**Volatility**

Volatility is the tendency of a substance to vaporize and is directly related to a substance's vapor pressure (pressure at which a gas phase is in balance with the condensed phase). The higher the vapor pressure, the more readily a substance vaporizes.

In Aromatherapy, essential oils that are most volatile are considered top notes. These are the oils that are the quickest to evaporate from a blend. Medium evaporating oils are called middle notes and the slowest essential oils to evaporate from a blend are called base notes. When making a blend, it is beneficial to include essential oils from the top, middle and base notes. This is accomplished by using a ratio formula of 3 drops of top notes to 2 drops of middle notes to 1 drop of base note (the 3-2-1) formula. You can also double your mixes by using 6 drops of top note to 4 drops of middle note to 2 drops of base notes (6-4-2). This type of blending isn't set in stone but it is a nice way to guarantee a more even and thorough blending, especially in perfumes.

**The Properties of the Notes**

- **Top Notes-**Top notes are light, fresh and evaporate quickly. It is the first scent that you are aware of in a blend and it is the first scent to leave the blend. Most of the citrus essential oils fall into this group.
- **Middle Notes-**Middle notes evaporate at a slower rate of speed and they are noted for adding stability to the top notes. The middle note is considered the body of the blend, and/or fragrance.
- **Bottom** Notes-Bottom notes are slow to evaporate. The fragrances of these essential oils are rich and full body. When used in a blend, the bottom notes take a while for the scent to emerge, but once they do, they can linger for a long time. Use essential oils from this category sparingly.

## Short Chart of Essential Oils and their Notes

| TOP notes | MIDDLE notes | BOTTOM notes |
|---|---|---|
| Basil | Bay | Balsam peru |
| Bergamot | Black Pepper | Cassia |
| Cajupet | Cardamom | Cedarwood |
| Clary Sage | Chamomile | Cinnamon Bark |
| Coriander | Cinnamon | Clove |
| Eucalyptus | Cypress | Frankincense |
| Grapefruits | Geranium | Ginger |
| Hyssop | Calendula | Jasmine |
| Lemon | Juniper | Myrrh |
| Lemongrass | Lavender | Neroli |
| Lime | Marjoram | Nutmeg |
| Mandarin | Melissa | Oakmoss |
| Myrtle | Myrtle | Patchouli |
| Niaouli | Palma Rosa | Rose |
| Orange | Pepper | Rosewood |
| Oregano | Peppermint | Sandalwood |
| Peppermint | Pine | Vervain |
| Petitgrain | Rosemary | Vanilla |
| Ravensara | Rosewood | Vetiver |
| Tea Tree | Spineward | Ylang Ylang |
| Thyme | Yarrow | |

## Basic Guidelines

When making the perfect blend, it is important to combine essential oils with high, middle, and base notes that complement each other. There are many ways of accomplishing this task. One way is work with a particular "family" of oils. One such family would be the citrus family; another would be the Wood family.

The citrus family of oils is notorious for being a "high" note which means that the scent of the oil disappears very quickly, making it very volatile.

The Wood family of oils tends to be more of the 'base' notes, or low notes making the scent of these oils last for a much longer time. Middle notes like Lavender and Geranium tend to make the top notes last longer, but it is the base notes that will dominate the blend if they are used in equal amounts with the middle and high notes. Here is a simple formula for you to remember when creating your next blend of essential oils:

## 3 – 2 – 1 to 1 ounce of carrier oil

The 3-2-1 blend stands for 3 drops of a high note, 2 drops of a middle note, and 1 drop of a base note added to 1 ounce of carrier oil. That is the basic blending formula to create the perfect blend. You can increase this basic formula to such degrees such as:

3-2-1
6-4-2
9-6-3
30-20-10

A typical recipe for making perfume is to use 25 drops of essential oil to 2 ½ ounces of carrier oil. This carrier oil can be pure grain alcohol, such as vodka, or you can just use jojoba oil. The 25 drops of essential oils that you will be using will still be based on the above 3-2-1- formula using 3 drops of top notes to every 2 drops of middle notes to 1 drop of every base note.

Fixatives such as Phthalates and Glycerin are sometimes added to the perfume to depress the evaporation rate of essential oils. Fixatives can come in either vegetable or animal while a wide range of synthetic substances are used today.

The problem with using Phthalates is that they are known to have a carcinogenic effect. Both Phthalates and Glycerin may cause or provoke allergic reactions in some people. Because of this fact, and the fact that essential oils do not evaporate very fast in the atmosphere, you may choose to leave fixatives out of your formulas, I know I do.

The important thing to remember though while you are creating your blends is KEEP NOTES! There is nothing like coming up with a wonderful finished product and then you find yourself unable to recreate it because you forgot the formula.

Another important thing to remember is that when your blend has time to sit for a while, it will change. The change may be ever so slight, but it will happen. It may even surprise and delight you. There is a lot of experimentation that goes on to create the perfect blend. With practice and patience, you will create a blend that is perfect and right for you, or your client.

**Synergies**

The effectiveness of any blend is dependent upon many factors. One such factor is the proportions of each essential oil used in the blend. This is vital to the effectiveness of the remedy as a whole. Some essential oils that are blended together have a mutually enhancing effect upon one another so that the whole is greater than the sum of the parts.

A good example would be the anti-inflammatory action of Chamomile which is supported by being mixed with Lavender. When blends work in harmony together, the combination is a "synergy," and every Aromatherapist wants to create a good one.

There are some things which should do in order to create a good synergy. One of these things is that you must take into account not only the symptom to be treated but also the underlying cause of the disorder, the biological, and the psychological or emotional factors involved.

This is why individual prescriptions are preferred over the mass produced "synergies" on the market today. Each blended essence is made for an individual's physical requirement, as well as, their emotional.

Essential Oils are also grouped together according to their common constituents such as camphoraceous oils containing a good percentage of cineol (members of the Mytacease group such as eucalyptus, tea tree, cajuput and myrtle.

Some essential oils such as rose, jasmine, oak moss and lavender seem to enhance just about any blend. Some combinations of essential oils have an inhibiting power over one another. You must learn the character of each essential oil before attempting blends with them.

It was a Frenchman named Piesse who instigated a new approach to classifying odors. He transformed the fragrances into corresponding notes. Together, these notes formed a balanced chord of harmony when blended together. Each essential oil is classified according to what Piesse believed to be that oils' dominant character.

## Temperature

Essential oils should be stored in dark, colored glass bottles away from direct heat sources, including a window sill where the sun can reach it. Store your bottles in a cool, dark place away from children and pets.

One place where you can store your citrus essential oils, as well as some of your carrier oils, is in the refrigerator. Be sure that your refrigerator is set between 5-10 degrees Celsius.

Refrigeration is not suggested for Aniseed, Fennel, Rose Otto, and Star Anise as these oils may solidify at cold temperatures. If this happens, you can still use the essential oil once you have let it warm back up at room temperature. Essential oils are flammable so be sure not to store them near stoves, fires, candles, or other sources of heat.

## Light

Essential oils should not be place where the sun can shine on it. If you place your essential oils where the sun can hit it, this will speed up the process called oxidation, which will deteriorate the overall effectiveness of the essential oil. Store all essential oils in dark colored bottles in a dark and cool storage place.

## Air

Essential oils are volatile which means that they will evaporate quickly when opened. Be sure to replace the cap quickly and tightly on your bottle of essential oil when you are finished using it.

The more often a bottle is opened, the more opportunities there will be for the properties of the essential oil to dissipate which will weaken the overall effectiveness of the essential oil.

**Space**

Another thing to notice is the size of the bottle that you are using in relation to the amount of essential oil left in the bottle. Always try to use the small bottle possible to house the most essential oil. This is because the empty space that is created by the amount left over in the bottle will encourage and hasten the speed of oxidation in the product. If you have only 2 ounces of essential oil left over in a 4 ounce bottle, then it would be beneficial to pour the 2 ounces of essential oil in a 2 ounce bottle.

**How to Detect Deterioration of an Essential Oil**

There are some ways in which you can notice if the essential oil that you are using has deteriorated. Look for cloudiness, thickening, or overall smell changes.

## Dilution Ratio

½% dilution for cats
1% dilution for children, pets and elderly
2% dilution for whole body massage
4% dilution for concentrated ailments

| Examples | Volume | 1% dilution | 2% dilution | 3% dilution |
|---|---|---|---|---|
| Room spray | 2 ounce bottle | 10 drops | 20 drops | 40 drops |
| Massage | 1 ounce bottle | 5 drops | 10 drops | 20 drops |
| Face mist | .5 ounce bottle | 3 drops | 6 drops | 12 drops |

Essential Oil Dilution Chart according to Bottle Size/Carrier Oil used

| Carrier | 1% # drops | 2% # drops | 5% # drops | 10% # drops | 20% # drops | 50% # drops |
|---|---|---|---|---|---|---|
| 5ml | 1 | 2 | 5 | 10 | 20 | 50 |
| 10ml | 2 | 4 | 10 | 20 | 40 | 100 |
| 30ml | 6 | 12 | 30 | 60 | 120 | 300 |
| 50ml | 10 | 20 | 50 | 100 | 200 | 500 |
| 100ml | 20 | 40 | 100 | 200 | 400 | 1000 |

Please note that anything more than 2% dilution should only be done by a trained Aromatherapist as they must be able to monitor their client carefully.

## Measurements (approximation):

1 ml...20-30 drops,
5 ml...1 tsp. or 1/6 ounce, 100 drops
10 ml...2 teaspoons or 1/3 ounces
15 ml...1 tablespoon or ½ ounce
30 ml...1 ounce or 2 tablespoons
60 ml...2 ounces or ¼ cup
120 mil...4 ounces or ½ cup
75 drops.......1 teaspoon
450 drops.....1 ounce
8 grams.........1 ounce
28.5 grams...1 ounce
3 teaspoons=1 tablespoon
16 tablespoons=1 cup
1 cup=8 ounces
2 cups=1 pint
4 cups=1 quart
4 quarts=1 gallon

## Equipment

Use only glass containers. Wear mask and gloves. Be sure you work in an open air environment so that you do not succumb to any fumes. Be sure to take notes of everything that you create so that you make it again.

**Chapter Eleven**
**Carrier Oils**

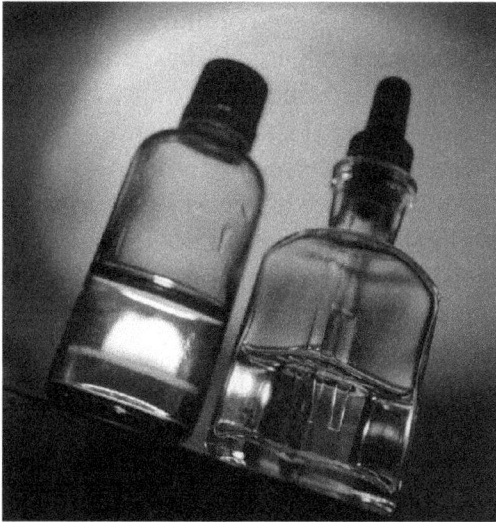

When selecting your carrier oils there are many things to take into account, how you will ultimately use the blend. Whatever carrier oil you use, remember that the properties of that oil will be added to your end product. For healing salves, I prefer to use olive oil to which I add Vitamin E to prolong the shelf life of the product. For creams and lotions, I am careful to discover the particular needs of the person who will be using the product. I take into consideration any and all contraindications that the user may have. For instance, if a person suffers from hay fever, I would not make them a product using Calendula carrier oils. Or, if a person was allergic to peanuts, I wouldn't use oil that contained nuts such as Sweet Almond, Hazelnut, Macadamia Nut, or Peanut Oil.

Following is a short list of carrier oils and their properties. There are many carrier oils to choose from but I have tried to list some of the most popular one below. For more information, please do more research by reading some of the fine books I have listed in the Reference section of this booklet. For massage purposes, use cold-pressed oils as they are absorbed more easily into the skin. Some good chooses would be sweet almond, sunflower, grape seed and coconut oil.

**List of some Carrier Oils**

**Aloe Vera**-(Aloe Vera)-Great for use in wound healing, sunburns, skin that is hot to the touch. Very cooling and refreshing.

**Apricot Kernel**-(Armeniaca vulgaris, Prunis armeniaca) - good facial oil; Vitamins A, B. Aids in healing/rejuvenating skin cells. Use on mature, dry and damaged skin.

**Avocado**-(Persea Americana, Persea gratissima) - good for dry, flaky, and aging skin types; rich and heavy with minor sunscreen effects. Expensive. Great to combine with other carrier oils in a blend. Oil is thick, rich and green in color. High in Vitamins A, D, E, lecithin and potassium (among others). Use on chapped hands, rashes, chaffing and even on babies for cradle cap.

**Baking Soda**-(sodium bicarbonate)-Used to absorb perspiration and odors, cleans carpets.

**Calendula oil**-(Calendula officinalis) - good as a body oil; speeds up healing/moisturizing for dry/damaged skin.

**Carrot oil**- (*Daucus carota L. var. Chantenay, fam. Apiaceae (Umbelliferae)*-Rich in Vitamin A and bet-carotene. Carrot oil can be used in conjunction with any skin healing essential oil blend. Use for liver disorders, gallbladder problems, hepatitis, colitis, ulcers and abscesses. Use for hair and skin tone, scars and acne. Great in anti-aging skin care products.

**Castor oil (Ricinus communis L)** - good for sealing in moisture; a heavy oil that seals and protects.

**Coconut Oil (Unfractionated)**-Use to moisturize and refresh skin. Easily absorbed into the skin.

**Colloidal Silver**-pure silver suspended in distilled water.

**Epson Salt**-(magnesium sulfate). Use to detoxify the skin, relieve sore muscles.

**Evening Primrose** – (Oemothera biennis)-antioxidant. Often added to other Carrier Oils to prolong shelf life.

**Grapeseed**-(Vitis vinifera) - good as a massage oil and facial oil; very light, penetrates the skin quickly. Slightly astringent (use for acne, oily skin), facial toner, cellulite, skin tightening. Relatively inexpensive.

**Hazelnut oil** – (Corylus avellana) - good for facials; loaded with vitamins, minerals and proteins. High Vitamins A, B, E and linoleic acid. Great skin absorption.

**Hemp-**(Canabis sativa)-reduces roughness and irritation. Good for cracked hands and feet.

**Jojoba oil-**(Simmondsia sinensis, Buxux sinensis) - very dry/oily skin; often added to other Carrier Oils to prolong their shelf life. Not an oil as such but a liquid was, makes this oil more stable than other oils and the first choice in making blends for resale (since they can have a shelf life of 10 or more years). Use for skin conditions such as rashes, psoriasis and eczema.

**Macadamia-**(Macadamia tenuifolia)-use for eczema, dry chapped skin, psoriasis and burns. This oil is rich in palmitoleic acid which is great for delaying the onset of skin and cell damage.

**Olive oil-**(Olea europaea) - "extra virgin" has the highest amount of vitamins and minerals. Great to use in homemade soaps and shampoos. Little thick so you can mix with other oils.

**Safflower Oil-**(Carthamus tinctorius Flos.) - good for softening the kin; it's a light-to-medium weight oil.

**Shea Butter-**vitellaria paradoza-Thick wax from Shea nuts for wound and skin healing.

**St. John's Wort-**(*Hypericum perforatum*)-also known as Hypericum oil is used for soft tissue injuries. Good to use for neuralgia, shingles, RA, and other ailments that result in pain in the nerve endings.

**Sunflower oil-**(Helianthus annuus) - good for massage, body lotions, and body oils; rich in Vitamin E. Cold-pressed sunflower oil is best to use as it contains essential fatty acids beneficial for skin healing treatments.

**Sweet Almond-**(prunus amygdalus, P. dulcis)-Great to use on dry and itchy skin. Also good for skin that is inflamed. Works well in massage oil blends. Sweet and lightweight.

**Vitamin E oil** - good for prolonging the shelf life of other Carrier Oils; very thick; Use in 10% dilution to preserve a blend. Antioxidant properties; heals scar tissue and rejuvenates skin cellular activity. Great for mature skin, scar tissue or stretch marks. Great source of unsaturated fatty acids and Vitamins A and E.

**Wheatgerm oil-**(Triticum saivum) - good for healing scars, burns and stretch marks; Vitamins A, D, and E

Please remember that a carrier oil can be anything that you put essential oils into which includes bath water, honey, dead sea salts, lotions, creams, gels, etc.

**Chapter Twelve**
**Essential Oils - 25 Specific Essential Oils**

**Essential Oil #1: Helichrysum,** known as *Everlasting Essential Oil* or *Immortelle*.
**Botanical Name**: Helichrysum italicum (everlasting or immortelle)
**Aromatic Scent:** Warm, earthy and bittersweet
**Plant Part:** Flowering Tops of Plant
**Extraction Method:** Steam Distilled
**Country of Origin:** Croatia
**Color:** Pale yellow
**Viscosity:** Thin
**Distillation Method**: Steam-distillation
**Blends well with**: Chamomile, Lavender, Clary Sage, and Rose.

**On the Emotional Level:** Use this oil to open the Heart Chakra, clear old emotional wounds, let go of grudges and resentments, learn to forgive others and to be forgiven. Use to unblock/regulate energy in the body, release of Qi (Chi), restore compassion.

**On the Physical Level:** Use this oil for healing the skin, scars and wounds. Release muscle knots, anti-inflammatory, chelation (use on soles of feet to remove metals from the body), tissue rejuvenation, burn healing, reduce swelling, back and neck pain reduction, reduce surgical scarring, use on arthritic conditions, dissipates free radicals, analgesic, supports liver function, use on areas for numbness and tingling. May also help those with hearing loss/damage or suffer from tinnitus (just place a drop of essential oil on cotton ball and place it in the ear while sleeping each night for two weeks).

**Caution:** For external use only. Do not use directly on skin, dilute in a carrier oil. If skin sensitivity occurs, discontinue use. If you are pregnant, nursing or taking any medications, consult your doctor before use.

**Essential Oil #2: Clove**.
**Botanical Name**: Eugenia caryophllata
**Aromatic Scent**: Sweet, spicy and penetrating
**Plant Part:** Buds, leaves or stems
**Oil Characteristics:** Anesthetic, antibacterial, antifungal, antiviral, antiseptic, anti-inflammatory, and antispasmodic, aphrodisiac. Antiparasitic, stimulant and vermifuge.
**Extraction Method:** Steam-distillation
**Country of Origin:** Molucca Islands
**Color**: Pale yellow
**Viscosity**: Medium
**Blends well with**: Roman Chamomile, lemon, lavender, sandalwood, peppermint, thyme, geranium, pine, ravensara, inula, ginger, eucalyptus, rose, frankincense, ylang ylang and citrus oils.

**On the Emotional Level:** Use this oil to help calm an overworked mind, nervousness, anxiety,, stress and tension, mental exhaustion

**On the Physical Level:** Stimulates a sluggish digestive tract,
Restores the appetite.
Relieves pain and arthritic joints
Relieves gas (flatulence) and bloating (when used in massage)
Relieve toothaches or combat gum infections
Use for neuralgia
Use for parasites

**Caution:** A dermal and mucous membrane irritant. May be sensitizing. May inhibit blood clotting. Contraindicated for those who are using blood thinners/ May irritate the liver with prolonged use.

**Essential Oil #3: Vetiver**
**Botanical Name**: Vetiveria zizanoides
**Aromatic** Scent: Earthy, hint of wood, sweet
**Plant Part**: roots
**Oil Characteristics**: antibacterial, antiseptic, calming, coolant,
   moisturizing, **nervine, sedative, tonic, vermifuge**
**Extraction** Method: Steam-distillation
**Country of Origin**: Tropical Asia
**Color:** Olive green to dark brown
**Viscosity:** Very thick to molasses like
**Blends well with**: Rosemary, rosewood, lavender, pine, patchouli, all
   citrus oils, chamomile, frankincense, ylang ylang, eucalyptus,
   rose, sandalwood, peppermint, oregano, thyme, pine and
   geranium.

**On the Emotional Level:** calms hysteria and neurotic behavior.
   Relieves mental exhaustion. Calms irritability. Calms frustration,
   anxiousness and nervousness. Relieves feelings of anger, stress
   and tension. Use for those who are absent minded and need
   grounding.

**On the Physical Level:** Elevates progesterone levels, Hormone
   balancing
         Helps alleviate PMS and menopause
         Use to relieve physical exhaustion
         Use for skin conditions such as acne, dermatitis, psoriasi,
         Use for arthritis

**Used as a fixative in cosmetics, perfumes and colognes**

**Caution: none**

**Essential Oil #4: Ginger**
**Botanical Name**: Zingiber officinalis
**Aromatic Scent**: Spicy, sweet and peppery
**Plant Part**: Root
**Oil Characteristics:** Analgesic, antiseptic, antispasmodic, antibacterial, antiviral,, febrifuge, stimulant, tonic and expectorant.
**Extraction Method**: Steam Distilled
**Country of Origin**: India, East Asia, Australia
**Color:** Clear to pale yellow
**Viscosity**: Medium to thick
**Blends well with**: All citrus oils, lavender, chamomile, frankincense, ylang ylang, eucalyptus, sandalwood, peppermint, rosemary, oregano, thyme, pine, garnaium, rose, jasmine

**On the Emotional Level:** Use for grounding. Helps with those who are frigid and emotionally withdrawn.

**On the Physical Level:** Use to relieve pain from arthritis and sciatica
Promotes menstruation while easing cramping, relieves hormone
headaches
Aid in memory
Aids in digestion, nausea relief
Use for fluid retention
Helps with dry coughs, colds and flu
**Caution:** May cause skin irritation

**Essential Oil #5: Sweet Thyme**
**Botanical Name:** Thymus vulgaris ct. linalol
**Aromatic Scent:** Fresh herbaceous aroma
**Plant Part**: leaves
**Oil Characteristics**: Antiseptic, antiviral, diuretic, carminative, antispasmodic, expectorant, antibacterial, disinfectant, stimulant, astringent, insecticide, febrifuge and antiparasitic.
**Extraction Method:** Steam Distilled
**Country of Origin**: n/a
**Color:** Clear to pale yellow
**Viscosity:** Thin to medium
**Blends well with**: All citrus oils, chamomile, lavender, frankincense, geranium, eucalyptus, myrrh, rosewood, sandalwood, vetiver, rosemary, oregano and pine
**On the Emotional Level:** Use for mental exhaustion.
**On the Physical Level:** Insect repellant
Mouthwash and gargle for sore throats or gum problems
Colds, flu, whooping cough, bronchitis, respiratory catarrh. Clears excess mucus from lungs. Use for asthma.
Digestive aid, flatulence. Use for gout and intestinal parasites.
Gastritis.
Epilepsy
Kills bacteria and airborne viruses.
Stimulates circulation.

**Caution:** too much can contraindicated for people with high blood pressure.

**Essential Oil #6: Inula (Also known as Elecampane) Inula helenium**
**Botanical Name**: Inula helenium; graveolens
**Aromatic Scent**: Sweet, mint-like
**Plant Part:** Flowering plant
**Oil Characteristics**: Antitussive, cardiac tonic, expectorant, mucolytic, refreshing, stimulation, antifungal, anti-asthmatic, anti-parasitic, analgesic, hormone balancing
**Extraction Method**: Steam Distilled
**Country of Origin:** Mediterranean region
**Color:** Emerald green
**Viscosity:** Thick
**Blends well with:** All citrus oils, chamomile, frankincense, lavender, ravensara, eucalyptus, sandalwood, peppermint, geranium, cinnamon, myrrh, rose
**On the Emotional Level:** Helps with mental instability.
**On the Physical Level:** Viral infections such as AIDS, rashes, shingles, herpes
Increases heart, lymph and respiratory circulation
Helps with gall bladder, intestinal and digestive issues
Supports and balances the nervous system and adrenal fatigue
Helps with bronchitis, throat and lung ailments and infections
Help with tachycardia, arrhythmia and cardiac fatigue
**Caution:** Skin sensitivity. Skin irritant.


**NOTE:** Elecampane was used by the Romans and Greeks as a cure-all and by the Anglo-Saxons for skin diseases.

**Essential Oil 7#:  Jasmine, known as the "Queen of the Night" in India**

**Botanical Name:** Jasminum officinalis

**Aromatic Scent**:  Sweet and Floral

**Plant Part**: Flower petals (picked before daylight)

**Oil Characteristics**: Analgesic, anti-depressant, aphrodisiac, antispasmodic, cicatrizant, euphoric, galactagogue, sedative, stimulant, uterine tonic

**Extraction Method**: Steam Distilled

**Country of Origin**: China, India and the Middle East

**Color:** Amber to dark reddish-brown

**Viscosity**: Thick

**Blends well with**: All citrus oils, chamomile, frankincense, lavender, ylang ylang, neroli, geranium, sandalwood, pine, bay laurel, patchouli, rose, helichrysum

**On the Emotional Level:** Helps with depression and mood swings.

**On the Physical Level:** Suppresses milk production

Helps with impotence, frigidity

Helps with insomnia, nightmares

Helps to stimulate uterine contractions during childbirth

Helps with postpartum depression, mood swings, hot flashes, PMS

Helps with irritability, stress

**Caution:** Avoid using this essential oil if you are a lactating mother as some sources believe it can stop lactation while other do not. Use Inula Sweet (inula Helenium) instead.

**Essential Oil 8#: Bay Laurel**
**Botanical Name**: Laurus nobilis
**Aromatic Scent**: Sweet, floral with a hint of clove and cinnamon
**Plant Part**: Leaves
**Oil Characteristics**: Anitbacterial, antiviral, analgesic, antiseptic, antispasmodic, emmenagogue, stomachic, tonic, febrifuge, sudorific, appetitie stimulant.
**Extraction Method:** Steam Distilled
**Country of Origin**: Mediterranean region
**Color**: Greenish-yellow
**Viscosity**: Thin to medium
**Blends well with:** All citrus oils, chamomile, frankincense, lavender, marjoram, rose, eucalyptus, sandalwood, peppermint, rosemary, helichrysum, pine and geranium
**On the Emotional Level:** Use for those who are afraid of being abandoned.
  Increases ESP. insight, intuition and inspiration. Use for people who feel emotionally withdrawn. Helps with those with depression.
**On the Physical Level:** Helps with pain
  Helps with respiration
  Helps to tonify liver and kidneys
  Helps to calm digestive issues
  Helps to protect against convulsions. Might help those with epilepsy and Parkinson's disease.

**Once used to crown athletes in the Roman times. A symbol of victory and wisdom**

**Caution:** May be skin sensitizing. Use in low doses on sensitive skin.

**Essential Oil 9#:  Lime**
**Botanical Name**: Citrus aurantifolia
**Aromatic Scent**: Sweet and tangy
**Plant Part**: rind, juice
**Oil Characteristics**: Antibacterial, antifungal, antiseptic, disinfectant, febrifuge, insecticide, tonic
**Extraction Method:** Steam Distilled from the juice –or- expressed from rind
**Country of Origin**: North America
**Color**: Clear
**Viscosity:** Thin
**Blends well with**: Citrus oils, basil, benzoin, bergamot, cedar, clove, coriander, eucalyptus, ginger, lavender, lemongrass, niaouli, parsley, peppermint, pine, sage, spearmint, spruce, tea tree
**On the Emotional Level:** uplifting, relieves stress, tension and anxiety. Helps fatigue, tired mind and spirit. Great to use when starting a new job, or moving to a new place.
**On the Physical Level:** Helps fight bacteria and fungal infections, including the common cold, flu and throat infections.
Use to move stagnant lymph, edema, cellulite and fluid retention.
Use for acne and oily skin
Use for cysts

**Caution:** Phototoxic

**Essential Oil 10#: Cedarwood, Atlas**
**Botanical Name**: Cedrus atlantica
**Aromatic Scent**: may smell like fresh cut timber
**Plant Part**: Wood
**Action:** Analgesic, anti-inflammatory, expectorant, sedative
**Extraction Method**: Steam-Distillation
**Country of Origin**: North Africa to Asia
**Color:** Pale yellow to dark amber
**Viscosity:** Medium
**Blends well with**: Other wood essential oils, lavender, rose, jasmine,
     pine, spruce
**On the Emotional Level:** Helps to reduce mental tension
**On the Physical Level:** Decreases blood pressure
     Helps with insomnia
     Helps with adrenal fatigue
     Helps with chronic respiratory problems (especially with mucus
       in the lungs)
     Helps with the allergic respiratory response by calming mast
       cells.

**Used in Tibet in incense and as medicine**

**Caution:** none known

**Essential Oil 11#:  Melissa (sometimes called balm and lemon balm)**
**Botanical Name**: Melissa officinalis
**Aromatic Scent**: Sweet and lemony
**Plant Part**: Flowering tops
*Oil Characteristics*: Antibacterial, antifungal, antimicrobial,
    antispasmodic, antiviral, sedative/
**Extraction Method:** Steam Distilled
**Country of Origin**: Europe and Central Asia
**Color**: Clear to pale yellow
**Viscosity**: Thin
**Blends well with:** Basil, roman chamomile, rose, geranium,
    frankincense, lavender, ylang-ylang
**On the Emotional Level:** Helps to alleviate depression
**On the Physical Level:** Combats the herpes simplex virus
    Use on Candida yeast infections
    Use for insomnia
    Use for headaches
    Helps with hypertension, anxiety and tense situations
    Helps with agitation due to dementia or Alzheimer's disease.
    Helps with spasms in the digestive tract (IBS) that is due to
        stress

**Caution:** Can cause skin sensitization. Do not use on people with allergies to ragweed.

**Essential Oil 12#: Fennel**
**Botanical Name**: Foeniculum vulgare
**Aromatic Scent**: Sweet and slightly spicy
**Plant Part**: Seeds
**Oil Characteristics**: antiseptic, antispasmodic, carminative, depurative, diuretic, emmenagogue, expectorant, galactagogue, laxative, stimulant, stomachic, splenic, tonic and vermifuge.
**Extraction Method:** Steam Distilled
**Country of Origin**: Mediterranean
**Color:** Clear to pale yellow
**Viscosity**: Thin
**Blends well with**: Geranium, lavender, rose and sandalwood
**On the Emotional Level:** Calms the nerves
**On the Physical Level:** Good digestive aid. Stimulates the release of bile from the liver
Use to detoxify the body
Use for gout, rheumatoid arthritis, cellulite. Use for kidney stones
Use as a tonic to strengthen after a bout of illness of exhaustion
In Europe, given to babies in a dilution of 0.5% in massage for colic
Use for PMS and menopausal problem (has estrogenic action)
Decreases appetite, aids weight loss, increases stamina
Use to promote lactaction and urination

**Caution:** Avoid if you have tumors or cysts that are estrogen based.

**Essential Oil #13: Basil, Exotic**
**Botanical Name**: Ocimum basilicum
**Country Grown**: India
**Viscosity:** Thin like water
**Actions**: Aphrodisiac, Insect Repellent, Uplifting, Anti-Depressant, Soothing, Antiseptic, Stomachic, Digestive, Tonic
**Characteristics:** Faint Licorice scent. Sharp and warm.
**Method: Steam** Distillation
**Note:** Top
**Physical Uses**: Energizing, elevating and anti-depressive
Use with children who have ADD and ADHD to help them focus
Clears a fogged head
Helps the Mind to focus
Helps with memory
Use when working on creative/intellectual tasks (like studying for test)
Bronchitis
Headaches and Migraines
**Emotional Uses**: Anti-Depressive, energizing, elevating
**Blends well with**: Eucalyptus, Geranium, Tea Tree, Lavender, Bergamot
**Contraindications:** Avoid during pregnancy. Could irritate or sensitize delicate skin. May irritate eyes. If irritation persists, call a physician, remove contact lenses and flush eyes with cool water for 15-20 minutes. Remove contaminated clothing and wash skin with mild soap and water.

**Essential Oil #14: Sweet Marjoram**
**Botanical Name**: Origana marjorana
**Country:** Hungary using the wildcrafted method
**Viscosity**: Thin like water
**Note:** Middle
**Actions**: Anaphrodisiac (reduces sexual desire) Respiratory problems, Warming, Tonic, Soothing, Relaxant, Antiseptic, digestive. Analgesic, anti-oxidant, antiviral, bactericidal, carminative, cephalic, cordial, diaphoretic, digestive, diuretic, emmenagogue, expectorant, fungicidal, hypotensive, laxative, nervine, sedative, stomachic, tonic, vulnerary
**Characteristics:** Warm and spicy
**Method:** Steam Distillation from flowers
**Physical Uses:** Use in a compress to relieve stomach and digestive problems
Use for insomnia sufferers
Use to reduce muscle tension
Use to reduce inflammation and spasms
Use for respiratory problems, asthma, colds and flu
Use to help balance blood pressure
Use to help relieve Arthritis and Rheumatism
**Emotional Uses**: Eases feelings of loneliness and rejection
**Blends well with**: Peppermint, Eucalyptus, Clary Sage, Lavender, Roman Chamomile, Bergamot, Rosemary
**Contraindications:** Do not use during pregnancy

**Use in soaps, detergents, cosmetic and perfumes**

**Essential Oil: #15: Siberian Pine**
**Botanical Name**: *Abies Siberica*
**Country:** Made from the needles in East Asia
**Viscosity**: Thin like water
**Note**: Top
**Actions:** Calming, Sedative, Uplifting, Stimulating, Bactericide,
 Deodorant, Anti-fungal, Purifying, Antiseptic
**Characteristics:** Fresh and Woodsy
**Method**: Steam distillation from tree needles
**Physical Uses**: Increases circulation
 Clears the head
 Calming and sedative
 Use to relieve rheumatic pains
 Use for chest infections, cold, sore throats, sinusitis
 Use for respiratory problems including the lungs, asthma,
 coughs, bronchitis
 Use for lice, scabies
 Use for excessive perspiration
 Use for urinary infection and cystitis
 Use for neuralgia
**Emotional Uses**: Uplift emotions during illness, fatigue, nervous
 exhaustion and stress
**Blends well with:** Rosemary, Tea Tree, Lavender, Lemon, Eucalyptus
**Contraindications:** May irritate or sensitize delicate skin

**Essential Oil: #16: German Chamomile**
**Botanical Name**: Matricaria chamomilla
> Also known as: Wild Camomile, True Camomile, Scented Mayweed

**Country**: Switzerland, Germany
**Viscosity:** Medium
**Actions:** Analgesic, Anti-anemic, Antineuralgic, Antiphlogistic, Antiseptic, Antispasmodic, Bactericide, Carminative, Cholagogue, Cicatrizant, Digestive, Emmenogogue, Febrifuge, Hepatic, Hypnotic, Nerve Sedative, Stomachic, Sudorific, Tonic, Vermifuge, Vulnerary
**Characteristics**: Oil has a warm and herbaceous scent.
**Method:** Steam-distillation
**Physical Uses**: Use as a tea for children who suffer from cramps and/or stomach aches.
> Helps with flatulence, gas, diarrhea, menstrual cramps, abdominal discomfort,
> Inflammation of the testicles, increases perspiration
> Use as a compress for inflamed eyes and conjunctivitis (soothing), hemorrhoids
> Use as a compress for skin eruptions (soothing) for itching, wounds
> Use in a tea to gargle for toothache
> Use as a face wash for healthier skin and as a hair conditioner (blonde hair) for a healthy shine.
> Fever, neuralgia, rheumatic pains

**Emotional Uses**: Soothing and sedative
**Blends well with:** Bergamot, clary sage, rose geranium and lavender.
**Contraindications**: Allergy to ragweed

**Essential Oil: #17: Lemongrass (vervaine)**
**Botanical Name**: Cymbopogon citratus
**Country**: (originally from India) Guatemala, West India, Madagascar
**Viscosity:** Thin
**Actions:** Antiseptic, analgesic, anti-depressant, antimicrobial.
antipyretic, astringent, bactericidal, carminative, deodorant, diuretic, febrifuge, fungicidal, galactagogue, insecticidal, nervine, nervous system sedative and tonic.
**Note:** Top/Middle
**Characteristics**: Lemony, dark yellow to amber and reddish
**Method:** Steam-distillation
**Physical Uses:** Relieves muscle cramps, tones muscles and makes them more supple when used in a massage oil, increases circulation
Diffusion can help with sore throat, laryngitis, soothes fevers,
Beneficial in treating headaches. Relieves jetlag and nervous exhaustion
Cellulite, colitis, indigestion and gastroententis
Fleas, lice and ticks, relieves excessive perspiration, athlete's foot
Use on acne, pimples, and oily skin as a skin toner
**Emotional Uses**: Uplifting
**Blends well with**: Thyme, basil, patchouli, ylang ylang, pink grapefruit, coriander, black pepper, clary sage, ginger, cedarwood, geranium, jasmine, tea tree, and coriander.

**Contraindications:** Avoid if you have estrogen fed tumors or cysts, may irritate sensitive skin,

**Essential Oil: #18: Mandarin Orange (Satsuma, Tangerine)**
**Botanical Name:** Citrus reticulata
**Country**: Italy
**Viscosity**: Thin
**Note**: Top/Middle
**Actions**: Anti-spasmodic, digestive, antiseptic, anti-depressant, anti-inflammatory, carminative, diuretic, cholagogue, sedative and tonic.
**Characteristics**: Amber to Orange in Color
**Method:** Cold pressed from ripe fruit peel.
**Aroma:** Citrusy, sweet
**Physical Uses**: Aids in secretion of bile
Calms children, calms coughing, calms panic attacks
Relieves muscle spasms
**Emotional Uses**: Calms emotion, Relieves depression. Sedative.
**Blends well with**: Geranium, clove, clary sage, roman chamomile, sandalwood, juniper, frankincense, myrrh, basil, petitgrain
**Contraindications:** Photosensitive

**Essential Oil: #19: Neroli**
**Botanical Name:** Citrus auranlium var. amara
**Country**: Italy
**Viscosity**: Thin
**Actions:** antidepressant, antiseptic, anti-infectious, antispasmodic, aphrodisiac, bactericidal, carminative, cicatrisant, cytophylactic, cordial, deodorant, digestive, emollient, sedative and tonic.
**Characteristics:** Pale yellow to light orange in color, citrusy. Sweet and floral
**Method**: Steam-distilled
**Note:** Top
**Physical Uses**: Calms anger, panic attacks, heart palpitations and headaches

Use in oil or bath to prevent post-exercise stiffness, relieves muscle spasms

Rejuvenate and regenerate the skin including scars and stretch marks

Used in perfumes, soaps and eau-de-cologne.

Insomnia, depression, anxiety, stress, relaxes a fearful or anxious mind, shock

Calms digestive tract, intestinal spasms, colitis, stomach cramps, diarrhea

Neuralgia, vertigo,

Use topically to rejuvenate skin, broken capillaries, scars and stretch marks
**Emotional Uses:** Relaxes the body and mind
**Blends well with:** Clove, cedarwood, sandalwood, ylang ylang, rosewood, lavender and all citrus oils

**Contraindications**: Avoid constant use if you have low blood pressure as it is sedating.

**Essential Oil: #20: Black Pepper**
**Botanical Name**: Piper nigrum
**Country**: India, Malaysia, Madagascar, (Singapore) China and
        Indonesia
**Viscosity:** Thin
**Actions:** analgesic, antiseptic, antispasmodic, antitoxic, aphrodisiac,
        diaphoretic, digestive, diuretic, febrifuge, laxative, rubefacient
        and tonic
**Characteristics**: Warm and spicy with a color from light amber to
        yellow-green.
**Method**: Steam-distillation
**Note:** Middle
**Physical Uses**: Increases warmth in body and mind, boosts the immune
        system (tones the spleen), and tones the digestive system.
        Stimulates the digestive system, the kidneys and circulation to
                the skin
        Relieves sore muscles and joints, exhaustion, fevers
        Pain relief, rheumatism, colds and flu, muscular aches, bruising,
                arthritis
        Stimulates appetite and encourages peristalsis, increases the flow
                of saliva
        Tones the colon muscles
**Emotional Uses**: Relieve coldness
**Blends well with**: Bergamot, clary sage, clove, coriander, fennel,
        frankincense, geranium, ginger, grapefruit, lavender, juniper,
        lemon, lime, mandarin, sage and ylang ylang.

**Contraindications:** May cause skin irritation. Avoid in pregnancy.
        May over-stimulate the kidneys.

**Essential Oil: #21: Citronella**

**Botanical Name**: Cymbopogon nardus (also known as Andropogon
nardus)

**Country**: Sri Lanka and Java

**Viscosity**: Medium

**Actions**: Antiseptic, bactericidal, deodorant, diaphoretic, insecticide,
parasitic, tonic and stimulant

**Characteristics:** Slightly sweet and lemony smell

**Method:** Steam-distillation

**Note:** Top/Middle

**Physical Uses**: Insect repellant, room freshener, candle wax,
deodorizing

Use in skin care products to soften skin, balance oily skin and
sweaty feet

Used in deodorants, perfumes, skin lotions and soaps

General toning effect on the body, balances perspiration, reduces
fever

Use to fight against colds, flu and minor infections (including
intestinal parasites)

**Emotional Uses**: Clears the mind

**Blends well with**: Bergamot, geranium, lemon, orange, lavender and
pine

**Contraindications**: Avoid if you have estrogen fed tumors or cysts.
May cause dermatitis. May irriate sensitive skin.

**Essential Oil: #22: Cinnamon**

**Botanical Name**: Cinnamomum zeylanicum (also known as C. verum and Laurus cinnamomum

**Country** Grown: Indonesia, Sri Lanka, India

**Viscosity:** Light to Medium

**Actions**: Analgesic, antiseptic, antibiotic, antispasmodic, aphrodisiac, astringent, cardiac, carminative, emmenagogue, insecticide, stimulant, stomachic, tonic and vermifuge.

**Characteristics**: Spicy warm and musky smell. Color is yellow to red-brown

**Method**: Steam-distillation

**Note**: Middle

**Physical Uses**: Helps the digestive (diarrhea) and immune system. Calms the nervous system.
Use to fight infections of the respiratory tract, colds, influenza, bronchitis, warts
Use to relieve pain in arthritis, rheumatism and menstrual cramps
Fights feelings of exhaustion and depression, stimulates the glandular system

**Emotional Uses**: Fights depression

**Blends well with**: Clove, coriander, cardamom, frankincense, ginger, grapefruit, lavender, rosemary and thyme

**Contraindications**: May cause skin irritation (especially to mucus membranes). Avoid during pregnancy. High dosages may cause convulsions.

**Essential Oil: #23: Dill**
**Botanical Name**: Anethum sowa - also known as Indian Dill
**Country**: South West Asia
**Viscosity:** Thin
**Actions:** Antispasmodic, carminative, digestive, disinfectant, galactagogue, sedative, stomachic and sudorific.
**Characteristics:** Pale yellow with grassy smell
**Method**: Steam-distillation
**Note**: Top/Middle
**Physical Uses**: Assists with digestion (eases constipation and flatulence), hiccups,
Promotes wound healing, helps with excess sweating due to nervous tension
Calms headaches, stimulates milk flow in nursing mothers,
**Emotional Uses**: Combats feelings of being overwhelmed in times of crisis and/or trauma. Eases the mind.
**Blends well with**: Bergamot, caraway, nutmeg, all citrus oils.
**Contraindications**: Avoid during pregnancy

**Essential Oil: #24: Thyme**

**Botanical Name**: Thymus vulgaris (also known as Thymus aestivus, T. ilerdensis and T. velantianus)

**Country** Grown: Southern Europe, the Mediterranean, Asia Minor, and Central Asia, and cultivated in North America

**Viscosity:** Thin/Medium

**Actions**: Antirheumatic, antiseptic, antispasmodic, bactericidal, bechic, cardiac, carminative, cicatrisant, diuretic, emmenagogue, expectorant, hypertensive, insecticide, stimulant, tonic and vermifuge.

**Characteristics:** Sweet herby smell and reddish-brown to amber in color.

**Method:** Steam-distillation

**Note**: Middle

**Physical Uses**: Helps with memory, concentration and focus.

Used in incense in Greek temples. Used in Egyptian embalming process.

Stimulates the lung and bronchia, helps with bronchitis, coughs, colds, asthma, etc

Warms arthritis, rheumatism, sciatica and gout, poor circulation

Muscular aches and pains, sprains; Helps cellulite and obesity and edema.

Strengthens the nerves, fights feelings of exhaustion and depression

Tones the lung against colds, flu, coughs, asthma, laryngitis, sinusitis, sore throats and tonsillitis, etc. Boosts the immune system. Helps against chills and infectious diseases. As a urinary antiseptic it helps cystitis and urethritis.

**Emotional Uses**: Combats depression and feelings of exhaustion.

**Blends well with**: Bergamot, grapefruit, lemon, lavender, rosemary and pine

**Contraindications:** May cause skin irritation. Avoid during pregnancy. Avoid if you have high blood pressure. Do not use in skin care products.

**Essential Oil: #25: Nutmeg**
**Botanical Name**: Myristica fragrans (also known as Myristica
     officinalis, M. oromata and Nux moschata)
**Country** Grown: Sri Lanka, Java and the Molucca islands
**Viscosity**: Medium
**Actions**: Antirheumatic, antiseptic, antispasmodic, carminative,
     digestive, emmenagogue, laxative, parturient, stimulant and tonic.
**Characteristics**: Warm and spicy with a musky aroma.
**Method**: Steam-distillation
**Note:** Middle
**Physical Uses**: Fights inflammations and rheumatic pain, muscular
     aches and pains
     Assists the digestive system (intestinal disorders) and
     reproductive system
     Stimulates the mind, heart and circulation. Revives people who
     have fainted.
     Fights gallstones, encourages appetite and averts constipation
     Regulates periods, strengthens contractions during birth
     Gas, nausea, diarrhea and chronic vomiting. Tones hair follicles.
**Emotional Uses**: Relieves frigidity and impotence
**Blends well with**: Black pepper, cypress, geranium, clary sage,
     rosemary and orange
**Contraindications**: Toxic in large dosages and may cause nausea and
     stupor. Avoid during pregnancy.

**NOTES:**

**Chapter Thirteen**
**Professional Issues**

**Documentation**

Documentation is the process of collecting written information from your client regarding their past and current health history and care. This is also called the Client In-take Form or the Consent Form. This document will create a picture of your client's overall health, as well as, a basis for the assessment session and future treatment plant. This is the beginning of collecting information for your client's records. If the client has other documentations, such as x-rays, list of prescription medicines they are taking, etc., I will make copies of them and place them in the client's files.

This information should all be place in your client's folder. It is important to keep proper documentation on your client, not only for liability issue should they arise, but also because of the Health Insurance Portability and Accountability Act (HIPAA). This Act makes it possible for your client to share their information between your office and other health care providers. This is the way professionals should handle their clients. I can't tell you how many times I went to a massage therapist and didn't fill out any paperwork at all. They have no idea what my contraindications are or any of my medical history at all. Either they don't care, or they haven't been trained properly to handle any issues, or they are just cheating the IRS out of money which they don't plan on claiming on their income tax.

For the therapist, the documentation process helps them to choose what modality they will use, what areas to avoid or focus on, and to make judgments on amount of pressure to use depending upon the current health and needs of the client. The information that you collect in the above process is also legal evidence that may protect you or your business from being sued. Documentation established professional accountability and decreases the liability risk by the information that your client shared with you and it supports your chosen course of treatment.

In addition to diminishing your liability risk, documentation also helps in payment reimbursement, future research gathering data, improves quality of care, and demonstrates that the therapist followed accepted standards of care.

This is why everything should be documented. I even document every bruise, and their location, when a client comes in before I start the treatment protocols. Because you will forget a lot of information after a client leaves and you don't see them for another week or month, or perhaps even longer. I once had a client come back to me stating that one of my therapists had given her a bruise during treatment. I pulled her file and was happy to see that the therapist was efficient enough to have documented the finding of the bruise before she began the treatment session and had asked the client about it. Then the client remembered having talked with the therapist about it. See, this is how documentation can protect you and your reputation.

## The Treatment Plan

The treatment plan is a course of action that outlines the steps that you, the therapist, will do to help your client achieve their health care goals. This plan can shift and change as your client improves, or worsens, as the case may be. But this too should be in writing and placed in your client's folder.

Another form of documentation, especially for massage therapists and body workers, is called SOAP notes. Soap notes are what I use in every treatment session and it has you documenting the 'subjective' 'objective' 'assessment' and 'plan.' How this is done is when a client comes in for treatment, you will write down everything that your client says is wrong with them (the reason that they come in to seek treatment) under the S-Subjective section. The next section deals with the O-Objective and this is where the therapist will write down their visual and palpatory findings, and results of any tests that they are having the client to (such as range of motion results).

The A-Assessment section deals with the physician's diagnosis (if there is one) and everything that the therapist did in the session. The last section is the P-Plan section which contains the treatment plan.

In this section, the therapist will write done the type, duration and result of the modalities and techniques used for the current issue, as well as, for future visits.

There are other variations to the SOAP notes. One other is the APIE which stands for Assessment, Plan, Implementation and Evaluation. There isn't one form of documentation that is better than the other one. You will have to choose which one makes the best sense to you and which one you will not have trouble in completing each client session. Remember, filling out these forms is as much for your benefit as they are for your client's.

Be sure to place the SOAP notes in your client's charts at the end of each session. I always review the client's charts, and my notes, when the client returns for a follow-up session. I do this well before the client arrives at my office. My first question to them would be to see how they responded to their last treatment session. I will note anything that they say to me in the current weeks' note.

## Client Records

Client records are considered the property of the owners at the facility where the client has come for treatment, no matter the therapist was who did the work on them. If the therapist, who does the work on the client, also owns the facility, then the records belong to the therapist.

All records are required to be kept in a locked file cabinet for at least 4-7 years (depending on what state you live in) from the date of the last client session. Be aware that you may be subpoenaed by a court of law to give testimony about your client, especially if they have been in an auto accident. Your records will then be used to paint a picture of your client's health care needs and what you have done for your client. So be sure that you keep your writing professional as many professions will be looking at them. I already know of three cases where this has happened and only two of them kept any notes at all.

## Scope of Practice

In order to legally practice aromatherapy in your state, you must check with local rules and laws regarding such practice. Since I live in the State of Florida, I can only tell you what the laws are in regards to practicing Aromatherapy at this time.

In the State of Florida there are currently NO laws that prohibit a person from using, promoting, selling, and otherwise teaching aromatherapy classes. The laws as they relate to having a business DO count though.

Laws as they govern business practices are the following: A business license with your city or county municipalities to operate a business (which means you must operate a business legally in an area specifically designed for the operation of said business), apply for sales tax number is applicable, follow proper advertising procedures (no wild claims or promises), etc. More of these issues are covered in detail in the Aromatherapy Business Plan course. There are also labeling laws that can affect the sale of your product and we will be discussing these a little later in the course.

**NAHA Policy Statement on Raindrop therapy**

The following information has been taken from the NAHA official website at, www.NAHA.org,

"One of the fastest growing new areas for aromatherapy is the Spa industry. Here essential oils and hydrosols are used primarily for esthetic, detoxification, massage and relaxation 'treatments'. As interest in the use of aromatics increases in this field the need for in-depth training in Aromatherapy for Spa practitioners also becomes imperative. Clients seeking treatments should consider the scope of practice to be expected from a Spa and / or Spa treatments and should carefully decide at what point health concerns require expertise available only from a professional Aromatherapist or other qualified health practitioner. In particular there is concern regarding cure-based treatments such as Raindrop therapy." For more information on this statement, please visit www.NAHA.org.

**Additional Education and Resources**

There are always new findings in the Aromatherapy industry and it would be extremely professional of you to keep abreast of new research findings. There are classes and workshops help all over the country, as well as new books being published.

For up-to-date information you can check the website at www.NAHA.org or www.CropWatch.org. As more information comes in, I will also try to post them on my website at www.AromaCareBooks.com

**Quality of Essential Oils**

Currently, there are no quality standards or governmental issues to authenticate or judge the quality or performance of essential oils. There is not one set of standards in the United States on which to base the quality of essential oils on. The flowers and plants that are used to make essential oils are grown all over the world. Each grower and manufacturer has their own set of standards, integrity and practices on how they grow, harvest and create the final product-the essential oil.

As a consumer of essential oils, it will be up to you to assess the quality of the oils that you purchase and use. But there are some things that you can do that will help you to ascertain what a good product would be. There are some regulating and certifying organizations that may help.

One such regulating board is the Federal Food and Drug Administration (FDA). Under this governmental organization we have the Federal Food, Drug and Cosmetic Act (FDCA) and the Dietary Supplement Health and Education Act (DSHEA). The FDA is responsible for regulating food safety, labeling, dietary supplements, cosmetics, food allergens, food preparations and foodborne illness, infant formula, nutrition, production information, recalls and consumer advisories, education resource library, and more. The FDA also offers specific information for people with cancer, HIV/AIDS, pregnant, older adults, diabetics, transplant recipients, infants and toddlers.

The FDA has placed essential oils under either the cosmetic or drug category depending on how the essential oil is intended for use. These two categories are regulated very differently.

As a drug, the FDA will have more regulations on the safety and quality of the essential oil and consumers would need a prescription to purchase them (which is why most essential oils are not considered drugs). An essential oil will generally fall under the cosmetic category along with foods and flavoring agents.

The Federal Trade Commission regulates claims made in advertising but not product labeling. The Consumer Product Safety Commission is responsible for room fragrance systems, odor control systems, deodorizers, etc.

The FDA does NOT define what it means when a product says that it is 'hypoallergenic.' The FDA also does not define what the words 'organic' or 'natural' mean. That is why you can see labels stating that a chicken is organic or natural (because the chicken itself is both of these in loose terminologies) but it could have been raised in a pen and given growth hormones. So it is up to the consumer to research the products that they are purchasing and using.

Should you experience a bad reaction to a cosmetic (or essential oil), then you should do the following:

Stop using the product immediately

Call your primary care physician to find ways to care for your reaction.

Report serious problems to the FDA by calling 1-800-332-1088 or file online at www.fda.gov/medwatch/report.htm.

**Understanding Cosmetic Labels**
- Read list of ingredients to see if it contains something that you are allergic to. (If a product doesn't list its ingredients-I don't buy it.)
- Read the warnings on the label.
- Read the tips (if they exist) on the label.
- Hypoallergenic does not mean that it won't cause allergic reactions.
- Words like 'organic' or 'natural' does not mean that the product is safe.
- Check the expiration date of the products that you are going to use. (If a product doesn't list an expiration date-then I don't buy it).

**The Law and Labeling**

If you market your cosmetics to consumers on a retail basis (stores, online, home parties, conferences, door-to-door, etc.), then they must meet ingredient labeling requirements under the Fair Packaging and Labeling Act (FPLA). We will discuss more on labeling later in the course.

According to the FDA's regulation of cosmetics under the Federal Food, Drug and Cosmetic Act, cosmetics must not be adulterated or misbranded and it must be safe for consumers under labeled or customary conditions of use. Any color additives to the product must be approved for intended use. Packaging and labeling must not be deceptive, and must meet ingredient labeling requirements.

Outside of color additives, the law does not require cosmetic products and ingredients to be approved by the FDA before they go to market. It is your responsibility to ensure that your products are in compliance with all laws and regulations that apply to them, including proper labeling and product safety.

Cosmetics include products that cleanse the body, change a person' appearance and make a person more attractive. Products in this category include makeup, lipsticks, nail care products, perfumes, colognes, deodorants, hair dyes, shampoos, makeup removers, moisturizers, etc. The FDCA defines cosmetics by their 'intended use.' Cosmetics include products that are created to be poured, rubbed, sprinkled, or sprayed on the human body. These products are made for cleansing, altering the appearance, beautifying or promoting attractiveness.

If a product is intended to affect the way a person's body work, or is used to treat or prevent a disease, then this product is considered a drug under FDA rules and regulations. The FDA will look at the claims that the company is making with their product to make a ruling. Some products can be both a cosmetic and a drug. Be aware that if you plan on marketing your product as a drug then it must have pre-approval by the FDA.

The FDA encourages all domestic and foreign cosmetic firms to register their product formulations with the Voluntary Cosmetic Registration Program (VCRP).

This is a voluntary request and submitting your product information to VCRP does not indicate FDA approval. Only cosmetics currently available on the market in this country are eligible for registration on VCRP. The Bioterrorism Act of 2002 requires that all cosmetic ingredients that are also classified as a food product must meet certain requirements to registration.

For those who are making cosmetic products in their own home, it is completely legal to do so as far as the FDA is concerned. You will have to check with you state and local zoning laws before you set up shop in your basement. As long as the environment that you are working in will not adulterate your products (like dog hair getting into the mix, etc.), then you should be fine. The Good Manufacturing Practice (GMP) is a list of factors that an FDA investigator would look at during an inspection. This list will help you to understand how products and ingredients should be handled in order to insure their safety.

**List of possible contamination (adulterated).**
- Microbial contamination
- Color additive misuse
- Using prohibitive ingredients
- Using restricted ingredients
- Using packaging whose composition may injure health
- Unwanted substances showing up in the product (hair, nail, etc.)

**Safety Data**
You can use safety data that is published on products from the manufacturer, wholesaler or that is published in scientific journals such as on PubMed, TOXNET and on governmental websites. The Cosmetic Ingredient Review (CPR) is a website that contains information on the safety of cosmetic ingredients. It is operated by industry-funded panel of scientific and medical experts.

**Does Aromatherapy fall under cosmetics or drugs?**

When fragrance products are advertised as helping to improve a person's well-being in a variety of ways such as 'strengthening the immune system,' then these fragrance products are known as *behavioral fragrances* or *aromatherapy* products. While perfumes are considered as 'cosmetics' by the FDA, claims that a scent helps insomnia, helps in smoking cessation, or prevent a condition or disease, will have

The FDCA defines a drug by its intended use in the diagnosis, cure, treatment, mitigation or prevention of disease. That will affect the structure or function of the body of a human being or animal.

But what happens when a product is both a drug and a cosmetic such as an antidandruff shampoo that both cleanses the hair and treats dandruff? These products include deodorants, antiperspirants, moisturizers, toothpaste that contains fluoride, etc., must comply with the requirement from both cosmetics and drugs.

Cosmetic products and their ingredients (except for color additives), do not require FDA approval. Drugs do require FDA approval before they can be sold to the public. In order to start the process of getting FDA approval you will have to fill out the New Drug Application (NDA) where you will confirm to a "monograph" (rules) for a particular drug category.

**Soap**

Soap is regulated a little differently with the FDA. The FDA defines soap as a product that is labeled, sold and represented solely as soap and whose bulk of the nonvolatile matter in the product consists of an alkali salt of salty acids and the product's detergent properties are due to the alkali-fatty acid compounds (FDA, 2009). In this case, soap are regulated by the Consumer Product Safety Commission, no the FDA.

If a product consists of detergents, alkali salts of fatty acids, and is intended not only for cleansing but also to cure, treat, prevent disease or affect the structure or function of the human body than it is regulated as a drug (or as both a drug and cosmetic).

If a product consists of detergents, alkali salts of fatty acids, and is intended only for cleansing the human body and consumers associate with it as soap, then it is regulated as a cosmetic.

Some fragrance products are added to products that are used on the body for treating or preventing disease. Under the law, these types of use are considered drugs, or can be considered as both drugs and cosmetics. Some examples of statements associated with therapeutic uses include, 'easing muscle aches' or 'relieving headaches.'

Massage oils that are intended to lubricate the skin are considered a cosmetic under the FDA rule. But if you claim that the massage oil that you are using will help to relieve muscle aches or reduce a headache, then it could be classified as a drug, or possibly as both a drug and a cosmetic.

### How is intended use determined?

There are many ways that one can determine the intended use of a product. They are as follows:

- The ingredients in the product may determine a product's intended use.
- The statement on the label of the product.
- The marketing claims that are made on the product.
- Consumer expectations of the product.

### "Essential Oils" and "Aromatherapy"

Even though people use the term, essential oil, to refer to certain oils extracted from plants, the FDA has no regulator definition for the word. Essential oils are commonly used in 'aromatherapy' products and depending on what the product is used for, will depend upon on whether it is classified as a drug, cosmetic or both.

### Fragrance Ingredients

In Aromatherapy, we don't consider or use 'fragrance' in our work. We generally use essential oils only. Fragrance is usually a synthetically manufactured substance that does not have any organic connections to it. The FDA does not require approval for fragrances as they are only seen as cosmetic ingredients. Those who manufacture or market cosmetics have a legal responsibility to ensure product safety and proper labeling.

Fragrance and flavor ingredients can be listed as such under U.S. regulations. Both fragrance and flavor formulas are mixtures of natural and synthetic chemical ingredients. The FDA requires a list of ingredients for products sold to the public but it will not force a company to tell its 'trade secrets.' One of the main chemical components in fragrance products is diethyl phthalate (DEP) and is considered safe for human health.

While the FDA has authority to require allergen labeling for food, it does not have the same authority to require allergen labeling for cosmetics. If you have a problem with allergies or sensitive skin, then you may want to choose products that are fragrance free.

## What about Setting Standards around the world?

Even though the United States has been lagging behind in setting standards for the quality of essential oils, other countries have moved forward. One such country is France who created the Association Francaise de Normalisation, otherwise known as the Association French Normalization Organization (AFNOR). The organization provides directives and standards for members of the European Union states for companies that wish to exchange good within Europe. Some of the topics that AFNOR deals with have to do with determining water content, chromatographic profiles, content of phenols, etc.

The United States Pharmacopoeia (USPC) brings standards for medicinal preparations and The National Formulary (NF) set codes for the inactive ingredients that are used in medicine. Today, USPS and NF merged to publish a book called the United States Pharmacopeia-National Formulary (USP-NF), "USP-NF Red Book."

The book provides the FDA with enforceable standards for the quality and strength of health care products. The three volume book contains standards for dosage forms, drug substances, medical devices, medicines and dietary supplements.

Each monograph will include that name of the ingredient, its preparation, packaging, storage, labeling requirements, specifications, tests and procedures for tests, stipulated length, quality and purity.

A       nother organization the deals with setting standards for essential oils is the International Organization for Standardization, (ISO).

The ISO is an independent, non-governmental organization that promotes the development of standardization in the areas of intellectual, scientific, technological, and economic activity. It also provides guidelines for the packaging, conditioning, storage, labeling, sampling and testing of essential oils. ISO is based in Geneva, Switzerland, and it is made up of members from 162 countries around the world. ISO began in 1947 and since then it has published more than 19,500 International Standards covering almost every industry including food safety and healthcare.

The quality of essential oils can be impacted by a variety of environmental factors such as:

Altitude the plant is grown in
Soil Conditions
Amount of Rainfall
Use of Chemicals
Use of Pesticides
Country that the plant is grown in

## How do I find quality essential oils?

The Internet lists literally thousands of sources where you can purchase essential oils. But how can you choose which company is legitimate and which oils are top quality? There are a few guidelines and considerations that can help you in locating some good quality oils.

Read the Label. Locate the name of the country where the essential oil comes from. Lavender should come from France, etc. Plants grown in different countries will contain different constituents due to soil, water and air differences. Harvesting and distillation practices may also differ in different countries.

Read the Label. Locate the Latin name of the essential oil that you are looking for to be sure that you are purchasing the right 'species.' Some oils have many different species associated with them and each has a different action.

Smell the oil. The old adage, 'your nose knows' holds true for knowing the difference between good quality essential oils and bad ones.

What's the cost? The real deal will always cost more than the bad ones. If the essential oil is cheap, then it probably is cheap.

Check the producer's statement of purity. Are they claiming that it is 100% pure? Are they guaranteeing the quality?

Does the producer offer information on the how the essential oil was harvested (such as wildcrafting, private farming, etc.) or if it is certified organic?

Did the growers use pesticides or other chemicals while growing the plants to make essential oils?

Are the essential oils processed in a clean facility using good quality standards? Have they been diluted or adulterated in the process? Is it a clean facility or do they pets or rodents running through them?

How are the essential oils handled? Do the people handling the oils wear gloves, masks, etc.?

Are the essential oils packaged properly? Essential oils should be put in dark, glass containers to prevent oxidation.

How are the essential oils stored? Are they properly sealed and then stored in an air-conditioned facility, or are the subject to heat, light or oxygen?

## Gas Chromatography and Mass Spectrometry (GC/MS) Testing

GC/MS is the industry standard for identifying different substances in a test sample. This test is used for drug detection, detecting explosives, security, analyzes the atmosphere of other planets, food, aromatic products, and in newborn urine screening tests for more than 100 genetic metabolic disorders. It can detect substances in luggage and on human beings which makes it valuable to forensic experts.

This process of identification began in 1950 when chemists discovered a way to use gas-liquid chromatography to identify substances. But this method proved crude and inefficient. Later, Roland Gohkle and Fred McLafferty developed a new machine that used a mass spectrometer as the detector in gas chromatography. While this worked better than its predecessors, the device was large and fragile and limited to the lab setting.

Twenty years later, an analog-to-digital converter was added to the mass spectrometer which allowed computers to store and interpret the results. By the 20th century, CG-MS machines are now faster and more efficient than ever before.

These machines are used to analyze soil, water and air samples, and in the regulation of food, agriculture and medicines.

This amazing piece of technology can locate each substance in a mixture. How this works is that an operator will dissolve a sample of the object to be analyzed in a liquid and injects that liquid into a stream of gas. The gas will flow through a tube that has been specially coated to catch the compounds as they flow through it. This coating is used to separate each of the substances in the mixture. Each substance will come out of the tube at a different time and when it does, it is ionized and gets an electric charge. An electric magnet is then used to separate the pieces based on their weight. A computer will then measure the pieces and compare them against a computer library of known compounds and makes a list of not only the names of all of the substances in that mixture, but also how much of each substance was in the mixture.

In Aromatherapy, the GC-MS can monitor for organic pollutants in the environment but it may have trouble identifying some pesticides and herbicides as they are too similar to other related compounds. It is however, extensively used for the analysis of such compounds as: esters, fatty acids, alcohols, aldehydes, and terpenes. GC-MS can also be used to detect and measure contaminants from spoilage or adulteration which may be harmful.


Below is the U.S. Governments Fair Packaging and Labeling Act

TITLE 15 - COMMERCE AND TRADE
CHAPTER 39 - FAIR PACKAGING AND LABELING PROGRAM
**§1451. Congressional Delegation of Policy.**
Informed consumers are essential to the fair and efficient functioning of a free market economy. Packages and their labels should enable consumers to obtain accurate information as to the quantity of the contents and should facilitate value comparisons. Therefore, it is hereby declared to be the policy of the Congress to assist consumers and manufacturers in reaching these goals in the marketing of consumer goods.

## §1452. Unfair and Deceptive Packaging and Labeling: Scope of Prohibition.

### (a) Nonconforming labels

It shall be unlawful for any person engaged in the packaging or labeling of any consumer commodity (as defined in this chapter) for distribution in commerce, or for any person (other than a common carrier for hire, a contract carrier for hire, or a freight forwarder for hire) engaged in the distribution in commerce of any packaged or labeled consumer commodity, to distribute or to cause to be distributed in commerce any such commodity if such commodity is contained in a package, or if there is affixed to that commodity a label, which does not conform to the provisions of this chapter and of regulations promulgated under the authority of this chapter.

### (b) Exemptions

The prohibition contained in subsection (a) of this section shall not apply to persons engaged in business as wholesale or retail distributors of consumer commodities except to the extent that such persons (1) are engaged in the packaging or labeling of such commodities, or (2) prescribe or specify by any means the manner in which such commodities are packaged or labeled.

## §1453. Requirements of Labeling; Placement, Form, and Contents of Statement of Quantity; Supplemental Statement of Quantity.

### (a) Contents of label

No person subject to the prohibition contained in section 1452 of this title shall distribute or cause to be distributed in commerce any packaged consumer commodity unless in conformity with regulations which shall be established by the promulgating authority pursuant to section 1455 of this title which shall provide that -

(1) The commodity shall bear a label specifying the identity of the commodity and the name and place of business of the manufacturer, packer, or distributor;

(2) The net quantity of contents (in terms of weight or mass, measure, or numerical count) shall be separately and accurately stated in a uniform location upon the principal display panel of that label, using the most appropriate units of both the customary inch/pound system of measure, as provided in paragraph (3) of this subsection, and, except as provided

in paragraph (3)(A)(ii) or paragraph (6) of this subsection, the SI metric system;

(3) The separate label statement of net quantity of contents appearing upon or affixed to any package -

(A)

(i) if on a package labeled in terms of weight, shall be expressed in pounds, with any remainder in terms of ounces or common or decimal fractions of the pound; or in the case of liquid measure, in the largest whole unit (quarts, quarts and pints, or pints, as appropriate) with any remainder in terms of fluid ounces or common or decimal fractions of the pint or quart;

(ii) if on a random package, may be expressed in terms of pounds and decimal fractions of the pound carried out to not more than three decimal places and is not required to, but may, include a statement in terms of the SI metric system carried out to not more than three decimal places;

(iii) if on a package labeled in terms of linear measure, shall be expressed in terms of the largest whole unit (yards, yards and feet, or feet, as appropriate) with any remainder in terms of inches or common or decimal fractions of the foot or yard;

(iv) if on a package labeled in terms of measure of area, shall be expressed in terms of the largest whole square unit (square yards, square yards and square feet, or square feet, as appropriate) with any remainder in terms of square inches or common or decimal fractions of the square foot or square yard;

(B) shall appear in conspicuous and easily legible type in distinct contrast (by topography, layout, color, embossing, or molding) with other matter on the package;

(C) shall contain letters or numerals in a type size which shall be

(i) established in relationship to the area of the principal display panel of the package, and

(ii) uniform for all packages of substantially the same size; and

(D) shall be so placed that the lines of printed matter included in that statement are generally parallel to the base on which the package rests as it is designed to be displayed; and

(4) The label of any package of a consumer commodity which bears a representation as to the number of servings of such commodity

contained in such package shall bear a statement of the net quantity (in terms of weight or mass, measure, or numerical count) of each such serving.

(5) For purposes of paragraph (3)(A)(ii) of this subsection the term "random package" means a package which is one of a lot, shipment, or delivery of packages of the same consumer commodity with varying weights or masses, that is, packages with no fixed weight or mass pattern.

(6) The requirement of paragraph (2) that the statement of net quantity of contents include a statement in terms of the SI metric system shall not apply to foods that are packaged at the retail store level.

**(b) Supplemental statements**

No person subject to the prohibition contained in section 1452 of this title shall distribute or cause to be distributed in commerce any packaged consumer commodity if any qualifying words or phrases appear in conjunction with the separate statement of the net quantity of contents required by subsection (a) of this section, but nothing in this subsection or in paragraph (2) of subsection (a) of this section shall prohibit supplemental statements, at other places on the package, describing in nondeceptive terms the net quantity of contents: *Provided,* That such supplemental statements of net quantity of contents shall not include any term qualifying a unit of weight or mass, measure, or count that tends to exaggerate the amount of the commodity contained in the package.

**§1454. Rules and Regulations.**

**(a) Promulgating authority**

The authority to promulgate regulations under this chapter is vested in (A) the Secretary of Health and Human Services (referred to hereinafter as the "Secretary") with respect to any consumer commodity which is a food, drug, device, or cosmetic, as each such term is defined by section 321 of title 21; and (B) the Federal Trade Commission (referred to hereinafter as the "Commission") with respect to any other consumer commodity.

**(b) Exemption of commodities from regulations**

If the promulgating authority specified in this section finds that, because of the nature, form, or quantity of a particular consumer commodity, or for other good and sufficient reasons, full compliance with all the requirements otherwise applicable under section 1453 of this title is impracticable or is not necessary for the adequate protection of consumers, the Secretary or the Commission (whichever the case may be) shall promulgate regulations exempting such commodity from those requirements to the extent and under such conditions as the promulgating authority determines to be consistent with section 1451 of this title.

**(c) Scope of additional regulations**

Whenever the promulgating authority determines that regulations containing prohibitions or requirements other than those prescribed by section 1453 of this title are necessary to prevent the deception of consumers or to facilitate value comparisons as to any consumer commodity, such authority shall promulgate with respect to that commodity regulations effective to -

(1) establish and define standards for characterization of the size of a package enclosing any consumer commodity, which may be used to supplement the label statement of net quantity of contents of packages containing such commodity, but this paragraph shall not be construed as authorizing any limitation on the size, shape, weight or mass, dimensions, or number of packages which may be used to enclose any commodity;

(2) regulate the placement upon any package containing any commodity, or upon any label affixed to such commodity, of any printed matter stating or representing by implication that such commodity is offered for retail sale at a price lower than the ordinary and customary retail sale price or that a retail sale price advantage is accorded to purchasers thereof by reason of the size of that package or the quantity of its contents;

(3) require that the label on each package of a consumer commodity (other than one which is a food within the meaning of section 321(f) of title 21) bear (A) the common or usual name of such consumer commodity, if any, and (B) in case such consumer commodity consists of two or more ingredients, the common or usual name of each such ingredient listed in order of decreasing predominance, but nothing in this paragraph shall be deemed to require that any trade secret be divulged; or

(4) prevent the nonfunctional-slack-fill of packages containing consumer commodities. For purposes of paragraph (4) of this subsection, a package shall be deemed to be nonfunctionally slack-filled if it is filled to substantially less than its capacity for reasons other than (A) protection of the contents of such package or (B) the requirements of machines used for enclosing the contents in such package.

**(d) Development by manufacturers, packers, and distributors of voluntary product standards**

Whenever the Secretary of Commerce determines that there is undue proliferation of the weights or masses, measures, or quantities in which any consumer commodity or reasonably comparable consumer commodities are being distributed in packages for sale at retail and such undue proliferation impairs the reasonable ability of consumers to make value comparisons with respect to such consumer commodity or commodities, he shall request manufacturers, packers, and distributors of the commodity or commodities to participate in the development of a voluntary product standard for such commodity or commodities under the procedures for the development of voluntary products standards established by the Secretary pursuant to section 272 of this title. Such procedures shall provide adequate manufacturer, packer, distributor, and consumer representation.

**(e) Report and recommendations to Congress upon industry failure to develop or abide by voluntary product standards**

If (1) after one year after the date on which the Secretary of Commerce first makes the request of manufacturers, packers, and distributors to participate in the development of a voluntary product standard as provided in subsection (d) of this section, he determines that such a standard will not be published pursuant to the provisions of such subsection (d), or (2) if such a standard is published and the Secretary of Commerce determines that it has not been observed, he shall promptly report such determination to the Congress with a statement of the efforts that have been made under the voluntary standards program and his recommendation as to whether Congress should enact legislation providing regulatory authority to deal with the situation in question.

**§1455. Procedures for Promulgation of Regulations.**

**(a) Hearings by Secretary of Health and Human Services**

Regulations promulgated by the Secretary under section 1453 or 1454 of this title shall be promulgated, and shall be subject to judicial review, pursuant to the provisions of subsections (e), (f), and (g) of section 371 of title 21. Hearings authorized or required for the promulgation of any such regulations by the Secretary shall be conducted by the Secretary or by such officer or employees of the Department of Health and Human Services as he may designate for that purpose.

**(b) Judicial review; hearings by Federal Trade Commission**

Regulations promulgated by the Commission under section 1453 or 1454 of this title shall be promulgated, and shall be subject to judicial review, by proceedings taken in conformity with the provisions of subsections (e), (f), and (g) of section 371 of title 21 in the same manner, and with the same effect, as if such proceedings were taken by the Secretary pursuant to subsection (a) of this section. Hearings authorized or required for the promulgation of any such regulations by the Commission shall be conducted by the Commission or by such officer or employee of the Commission as the Commission may designate for that purpose.

**(c) Cooperation with other departments and agencies**

In carrying into effect the provisions of this chapter, the Secretary and the Commission are authorized to cooperate with any department or agency of the United States, with any State, Commonwealth, or possession of the United States, and with any department, agency, or political subdivision of any such State, Commonwealth, or possession.

**(d) Returnable or reusable glass containers for beverages**

No regulation adopted under this chapter shall preclude the continued use of returnable or reusable glass containers for beverages in inventory or with the trade as of the effective date of this Act, nor shall any regulation under this chapter preclude the orderly disposal of packages in inventory or with the trade as of the effective date of such regulation.

### §1456. Enforcement.

**(a) Misbranded consumer commodities**

Any consumer commodity which is a food, drug, device, or cosmetic, as each such term is defined by section 201 of the Federal Food, Drug, and Cosmetic Act (21 U.S.C. 321), and which is introduced or delivered for introduction into commerce in violation of any of the provisions of this chapter, or the regulations issued pursuant to this chapter, shall be

deemed to be misbranded within the meaning of chapter III of the Federal Food, Drug, and Cosmetic Act (21 U.S.C. 331 et seq.), but the provisions of section 303 of that Act (21 U.S.C. 333) shall have no application to any violation of section 1452 of this title.

**(b) Unfair or deceptive acts or practices in commerce**

Any violation of any of the provisions of this chapter, or the regulations issued pursuant to this chapter, with respect to any consumer commodity which is not a food, drug, device, or cosmetic, shall constitute an unfair or deceptive act or practice in commerce in violation of section 45(a)of this title and shall be subject to enforcement under section 45(b) of this title.

**(c) Imports**

In the case of any imports into the United States of any consumer commodity covered by this chapter, the provisions of sections 1453 and 1454 of this title shall be enforced by the Secretary of the Treasury pursuant to section 801(a) and (b) of the Federal Food, Drug, and Cosmetic Act (21 U.S.C. 381).

### §1457. Annual Reports to Congress: Submission Dates.

Each officer or agency required or authorized by this chapter to promulgate regulations for the packaging or labeling of any consumer commodity, shall transmit to the Congress each year a report containing a full and complete description of the activities of that officer or agency for the administration and enforcement of this chapter during the preceding fiscal year. All agencies except the Department of Health and Human Services and the Federal Trade Commission shall submit their reports in January of each year. The Department of Health and Human Services shall include this report in its annual report to Congress on activities under the Federal Food, Drug, and Cosmetic Act (21 U.S.C. 301 et seq.), and the Federal Trade Commission shall include this report in the Commission's annual report to Congress.

### §1458. Cooperation with State Authorities; Transmittal of Regulations to States; Noninterference with Existing Programs.

(a) A copy of each regulation promulgated under this chapter shall be transmitted promptly to the Secretary of Commerce, who shall (1) transmit copies thereof to all appropriate State officers and agencies, and (2) furnish to such State officers and agencies information and

assistance to promote to the greatest practicable extent uniformity in State and Federal regulation of the labeling of consumer commodities.

(b) Nothing contained in this section shall be construed to impair or otherwise interfere with any program carried into effect by the Secretary of Health and Human Services under other provisions of law in cooperation with State governments or agencies, instrumentalities, or political subdivisions thereof.

### §1459. Definitions.

For the purpose of this chapter -

(a) The term "consumer commodity", except as otherwise specifically provided by this subsection, means any food, drug, device, or cosmetic (as those terms are defined by the Federal Food, Drug, and Cosmetic Act (21 U.S.C. 301 et seq.)), and any other article, product, or commodity of any kind or class which is customarily produced or distributed for sale through retail sales agencies or instrumentalities for consumption by individuals, or use by individuals for purposes of personal care or in the performance of services ordinarily rendered within the household, and which usually is consumed or expended in the course of such consumption or use. Such term does not include -

(1) any meat or meat product, poultry or poultry product, or tobacco or tobacco product;

(2) any commodity subject to packaging or labeling requirements imposed by the Secretary of Agriculture pursuant to the Federal Insecticide, Fungicide, and Rodenticide Act (7 U.S.C. 136 et seq.), or the provisions of the eighth paragraph under the heading "Bureau of Animal Industry" of the Act of March 4, 1913 (21 U.S.C. 151 et seq.), commonly known as the Virus-Serum-Toxin Act;

(3) any drug subject to the provisions of section 503(b)(1) or 506 of the Federal Food, Drug, and Cosmetic Act (21 U.S.C. 353(b)(1) and 356);

(4) any beverage subject to or complying with packaging or labeling requirements imposed under the Federal Alcohol Administration Act (27 U.S.C. 201 et seq.); or

(5) any commodity subject to the provisions of the Federal Seed Act (7 U.S.C. 1551 et seq.).

(b) The term "package" means any container or wrapping in which any consumer commodity is enclosed for use in the delivery or display of that consumer commodity to retail purchasers, but does not include -

(1) shipping containers or wrappings used solely for the transportation of any consumer commodity in bulk or in quantity to manufacturers, packers, or processors, or to wholesale or retail distributors thereof;

(2) shipping containers or outer wrappings used by retailers to ship or deliver any commodity to retail customers if such containers and wrappings bear no printed matter pertaining to any particular commodity; or

(3) containers subject to the provisions of the Act of August 3, 1912 (37 Stat. 250, as amended; 15 U.S.C. 231-233), or the Act of March 4, 1915 (38 Stat. 1186, as amended; 15 U.S.C. 234-236)

(c) The term "label" means any written, printed, or graphic matter affixed to any consumer commodity or affixed to or appearing upon a package containing any consumer commodity.

(d) The term "person" includes any firm, corporation, or association.

(e) The term "commerce" means (1) commerce between any State, the District of Columbia, the Commonwealth of Puerto Rico, or any territory or possession of the United States, and any place outside thereof, and (2) commerce within the District of Columbia or within any territory or possession of the United States not organized with a legislative body, but shall not include exports to foreign countries.

(f) The term "principal display panel" means that part of a label that is most likely to be displayed, presented, shown, or examined under normal and customary conditions of display for retail sale.

## §1460. Savings Provisions.

Nothing contained in this chapter shall be construed to repeal, invalidate, or supersede -

(a) the Federal Trade Commission Act (15 U.S.C. 41 et seq.) or any statute defined therein as an antitrust Act;

(b) the Federal Food, Drug, and Cosmetic Act (21 U.S.C. 301 et seq.); or

(c) the Federal Hazardous Substances Labeling Act (15 U.S.C. 1261 et seq.).

## §1461. Effect Upon State Law.

It is hereby declared that it is the express intent of Congress to supersede any and all laws of the States or political subdivisions thereof insofar as they may now or hereafter provide for the labeling of the net quantity of contents of the package of any consumer commodity covered by this chapter which are less stringent than or require information different from the requirements of section 1453 of this title or regulations promulgated pursuant thereto.

## §1451 note Effective Date.

Section 13 of Pub. L. 89-755 provided that: "This Act (enacting this chapter) shall take effect on July 1, 1967: Provided, That the Secretary (with respect to any consumer commodity which is a food, drug, device, or cosmetic, as those terms are defined by the Federal Food, Drug, and Cosmetic Act) (section 301 et seq. of Title 21, Food and Drugs), and the Commission (with respect to any other consumer commodity) may by regulation postpone, for an additional twelve-month period, the effective date of this Act (this chapter) with respect to any class or type of consumer commodity on the basis of a finding that such a postponement would be in the public interest."

11. Can I use a Post Office (P.O.) box or website for the address on the label?

A post office box or website address is not adequate for this labeling requirement.

The FD&C Act requires cosmetic labels to identify the name and place of business of the manufacturer, packer, or distributor. By regulation, this includes the street address, city, state, and ZIP code, although you may omit the street address if your firm is listed in a current city or telephone directory. You may use the main place of business instead of the actual place where the cosmetic was manufactured, packed, or distributed, unless such a statement would be misleading.

If you use the distributor's address, you must use a phrase such as "Distributed by" or "Manufactured for," followed by that firm's name and place of business. The name of the firm must be the corporate name. See the regulation on name and place of business at 21 CFR 701.12.

12. Where can I learn more about labeling requirements?

We can respond to specific labeling questions, but cosmetic labeling is not subject to premarket approval by FDA. It's your responsibility to make sure your labeling meets all requirements.

**Here are some useful resources**:

(b) Cosmetic Labeling and Label Claims: An overview to help you get started

(c) Cosmetic Labeling Guide: For step-by-step help that answers many common questions

(d) Cosmetic Labeling Regulations: For links to the full text of the regulations that apply to cosmetic labeling

(e) Some cosmetic labeling requirements are regulated by other federal agencies. For example, the U.S. Federal Trade Commission regulates claims of "Made in USA." Other country of origin labeling is regulated by U.S. Customs and Border Protection (see"Chapter 13-Country of Origin Marking").

(f) You may wish to work with a labeling consultant. FDA, as a government agency, does not provide referrals to private consultants. You may, however, find useful resources under "Trade and Professional Associations of Interest to the Cosmetic Industry" and "Cosmetic Trade Publications."

**Harvesting Practices and Procedures**

Another thing that affects the quality of essential oils is the harvesting practices and procedures that were followed in producing the essential oil. Some harvesting practices can add different chemical constituents to the essential oil over other practices that could be used to create the same essential oil elsewhere.

Harvesting methods also affect the oil yield and quality. If a plant is harvested at the wrong time of day (or season) the essential oils which are located in the oil glands/veins of the plant, may reduce the amount and quality of the essential oil. An example of this would be the harvesting of cinnamon bark. Normally, the cinnamon bark is harvested during the wet season when the rains have started peeling the bark. Harvesting takes place in the morning before the sun starts to dry out the bark.

## Ethics

Ethics is a system of moral principles as it relates to an individual and to a branch of philosophy that deals with the values and conduct of human beings. It is also seen as a rule of conduct in respect to a particular class of humans or groups such as medical ethics or business ethics. Ethics can also deal with actions that are seen as being either 'right' or 'wrong' and 'good' or 'bad.'

Many regulating and professional organizations will have a 'code of ethics' to which its membership must adhere to. This code of ethics is a set of guiding moral principles that is set out to govern the individual's course of action. A failure to do so would result in the organization to take action against the individual by either reprimand, loss of membership and even loss of licensure.

The code of ethics is important to any profession as it speaks to the integrity of both the group and the individual. Most of these codes include verbiage on honesty, anti-discriminatory procedures, confidentiality, professional boundaries, quality of care, scope of practice, informed consent, sexual contact, standards of practice and ethical decision making.

## Ethical Decision Making

When a client comes to you for help, they are putting themselves in a place of trust. You must respect trust relationship and do your best in making decisions concerning the health of your client. Not only must you be respectful of this imbalance of power, but you must also be ethical. The client has put their trust in you and your knowledge to help them with an issue.

You must make sure that the decision that you make for them (such as a course of treatment), is in their best interest and will not injure or harm them.

## Referrals

If you find that you client could benefit from a modality, or course of treatment, that is outside of your scope of practice or abilities, then you should give them a referral. This is not only the professional thing to do; it is the ethical thing to do.

The only problem with referring a client to another profession is if you get a kick-back from that professional. If you do receive something in exchange for the referral, then you run the risk of breaking the law in the United States.

Please be aware that if you give your client the name of another therapist, then you must also give them at least two other names of therapists in the same field. This is the law. The law that I am mentioning here is called the Stark and Anti-Kickback law that regulates the relationship between physicians and other healthcare providers.

The purpose of the law was to prevent physicians (and other healthcare providers) from referring a patient for certain services and then receiving a reimbursement for the referral. The act was meant to stop unnecessary testing. Violation of this law may result in a monetary penalty of up to $15,000 per violation and $100,000 per arrangements or overall scheme.

The Anti-Kickback Statute is a criminal statute that prohibits the willful solicitation or acceptance of any type of remuneration to induce referrals for health services. Remuneration includes savings on rental space (or free rent), percentage of client payments, free services, free education, or any other perks. Violations of this statute may result in a monetary penalty of up to $50,000 per violation.

## Prescription vs. Referral Form

A prescription is a written order from a physician or nurse practitioner authorizing a specific treatment. These orders are written on the physicians prescription pad and should include date, client's name, diagnosis and code, treatment order, frequency of treatments, duration of treatments and referring health care provider's name, signature and contact information.

Prescriptions are usually given for medication, therapy, or therapeutic devices. If a therapist accepts a prescription for therapy, then you provide ONLY what is listed on the prescription and be sure to document your service for the referring healthcare professional. The client would then return to the referring health care provider for their follow-up and evaluation. Therapist should retain the original prescription and add it to the client's file.

You can make copies for the client or referring physician, or for the insurance company, but you should always retain the original copy for yourself.

A referral form is generally produced by the healthcare provider (which can be you), and is given to and filled out by, the health care provider authorizing a specific treatment. These forms can contain the information listed above (except for the diagnosing part if you are not qualified to diagnose a condition).

**Code of Ethics**

The following is the Code of Ethics from the National Association of Holistic Aromatherapy (NAHA).

1.1 Demonstrate commitment to provide the highest quality aromatherapy service to those who seek their professional service

1.2 Conduct myself in a professional and ethical manner in relation to my clients, fellow aromatherapists & colleagues and the general public so as to comply with the highest standards of moral behavior & integrity and to uphold the dignity and status of my profession under all circumstances.

1.3 Share professional knowledge, research, and experiences with fellow aromatherapists and colleagues to support the advancement of aromatherapy.

1.4 Treat clients in accordance with holistic principles (Recommend treatment based upon the specific needs of the client.) and render professional services for no other purposes than the total well-being of my clients.

1.5 Educate clients in the quality and availability of true aromatherapy products and services.

1.6 Refrain from engaging in any sexual conduct or sexual activities involving clients.

1.7 Recognize that my primary obligation is always to the client and agree to practice Aromatherapy to the best of my ability for my client's benefit. My client's comfort, welfare and health must always have priority.

1.8 Provide clients with informed consent/disclosure statement and information that includes training, certification, scope of practice, payment structure, benefits, limitations and expectations of both the practitioner and client.

1.9 Endeavor to serve the best interests of my clients at all times by providing the highest quality of service and I shall undertake continuing education and improve upon my Aromatherapy skills and professional standards whenever possible.

1.10 Provide services within the scope and the limits of my training. I will not employ techniques for which I have not had adequate training and shall represent my education, training, qualifications and abilities honestly. I shall acknowledge the limitations of my skills and when necessary, refer clients to the appropriate qualified professionals.

1.11 Not diagnose, prescribe or provide any service, which requires a license to practice unless specifically licensed to do.

1.12 Maintain client confidentiality and not divulge to anyone the findings I acquire during consultation, or in the course of professional recommendations, without my clients consent except when required by law.

1.13 Support other Consultants at all time and shall never criticize, condemn or otherwise denigrate other Consultants in the presence of a client or other lay persons.

1.14 Respect the rights of other healthcare professionals and aromatherapists and will cooperate with all health care professionals in a friendly and professional manner.

1.15 Where another Consultant refers a client to me, I shall return such clients to the original Consultant when the specified recommendation is completed. I will not denigrate another Consultants recommendations.

1.16 Not make false claims regarding the potential benefits of Aromatherapy and shall actively participate in educating the public regarding the actual benefits of True Aromatherapy.

1.17 Not give guarantees regarding the results of any recommendations, nor exploit a client for financial gain through inferences or misrepresentation of any sort.

1.18 Practice honesty in advertising, promote my services ethically and in good taste, and practice and or advertise only those skills for which I have received adequate training or certification.

1.19 Maintain my premises in a hygienic condition, and ensure that my premises offer my Clients sufficient privacy.

1.20 Maintain complete records of each Client, including specific details of my recommendations.

1.21 Refrain from the use of any mind-altering drugs, alcohol, or intoxicants prior to or during a professional Aromatherapy consultation or while representing the National Association for Holistic Aromatherapy.

1.22 Dress in a professional manner, proper dress being defined as the attire suitable and consistent with accepted professional practice.

1.23 Represent a united front to the public and refrain from criticism of colleagues either in writing or verbally before clients or the general public.

1.24 Shall, upon being found to have transgressed any of the By-laws of the National Association for Holistic Aromatherapy and/or this Code of Ethics voluntarily surrender and return my membership certificate to the Association.

**NOTES:**

**Chapter Fourteen**
**How to make your Blend**


**Worksheet**
Begin with your bottle (choose dark or colored glass whenever possible).

Decide the purpose of your blend and write it down (i.e. relaxing, healing, chest rub, aching muscle massage lotion, etc.)

Make a list of the essential oils that will help with the purpose of the blend. Give priority to the list of essentials oils

Make a list of all of the carrier oils that will help with the purpose of the blend. Give priority to the list of carrier oils

Cross out all essential oils that will be contraindicated for your client.

Cross out all carrier oils that will be contraindicated for your client.

Narrow down your choice of essential oils to five or less (my preference).

Narrow down your choice of carrier oil to five or less (my preference).

Decide how much of a blend, or how many bottles, you are going to make.


If you are going to use more than 3 different essential oils, than look over the chart of top, middle and bottom notes and make a 3-2-1 ratio from your list of essential oils. (I generally never use more than 5 different essential oils in a blend). For every 1 drop of Bottom Note you will use 2 drops of Middle Notes and 3 drops of Top Notes. **NOTE**: I only use the 3-2-1- blending method if I am making products for resale.

If the product that I am using is going to be used up quickly, then I do not bother with it.

Calculate the drops of each of the oils per liquid that you will use. Are you using enough top, middle, and bottom notes? Are you making a blend in a particular family?

Begin by filling your chose bottle, or bottles, with the carrier oils that you have chosen. Keep notes on how much of each carrier oil that you are using.

Begin creating your blend by placing a drop of essential oil in the carrier liquid you are using and shake and smell. Continue to add drops of essential oils slowly, shaking and smelling often. Remember-you can always ADD more essential oils if you need to, but you can't the extra essential oils out of the blend once you have put them in. So be cautious. Take careful notes along the way.

After filling the container with your essential sniff it to see if it is pleasing and that you resonate with it. If you feel finished, then add the carrier oil, put the lid on the container and shake gently to blend.

Be sure to write on a piece a paper (or on a label for the container) the following information:

Name of the blend

Name of carrier oil(s) and essential oil(s) used

How many drops of each essential oil and carrier oil that was used (this information can be place in a notebook for your own private information if you prefer).

Date the blend

Put methods of application on the label (i.e. rube 3 drops on the soles of the feet before bed).

Put frequency of use on label (i.e. use twice a day).


## Additional Blending information and tips

Be sure to keep count of how many drops you use in your blend-write it down. This way you will be able to recreate your blend again.

Different carrier oils will take different amounts of essential oil. Sea salts will not require as much essential oils as distilled water will.

Massage oils are thicker than water so they do not require as much essential oils.

When you are creating your blend, be sure to take into consideration the properties of the carrier oil that you are using. If you are making a moisturizing blend you would NOT use Epson or sea salts as that would dry out the skin.

Be careful with essential oils as they will stain clothes and furniture.

Look over contraindications before creating a blend for yourself or others.

**Choosing your Carrier Oils according to your Skin Type**

<u>**Oily Skin**</u>

Skin can use the healing effects of the slightly more astringent yet balancing oils that will not plus up pores or make the condition worse. These are: Coconut Oil, Grapeseed, Hazelnut, and Jojoba

<u>**Mature Skin**</u>

The following oils are chosen because of their gentle and rejuvenating properties: Jojoba, Calendula, Rose Hip Seed, and Sea Buckthorn Berry.

<u>**All Skin**</u>

The following are carrier oils helpful to all skin types.

**Sweet Almond Oil** - relieves itching, soreness, dryness, and inflammation. This oil makes a good massage oil. Goes rancid quickly. Good for burns and thread veins. Very lubricating. Contains glycosides, minerals, vitamins A, B1, B2, B6 and E. Rich in protein.

**Apricot Kernel Oil** - Very rich and nourishing. Helpful for prematurely aged, sensitive, inflamed delicate or dry skin. Contains Minerals and Vitamins.

**Avocado Oil** - Very penetrating and nourishing for dry and dehydrated skin. Use for eczema, solar keratosis and to improve skin elasticity. A very thick and heavy oil.

Contains Vitamins A, B1, B2, D, E, Pahtothenic acid, protein, lecithen and fatty acids.

**Borage Seed Oil** - Use externally for psoriasis, eczema, prematurely aged skin, and to regenerate and stimulate skin cell activity. Contains Gamma Linolenic Acid, vitamins and minerals.

**Castor Oil** - Used to dissolve cysts, growths, warts, soften corns/calluses. Helps prevent scars. Helps dry, chapped skin and hair. Contains glyceride of ricinoleac, iso-ricinoleas, and stearic, linoleic and dehydroxysteric acids. Use as poultice

**Fractionated Coconut Oil** - Ideal for troubled skin and will not plug pores. Contains unrefined 50% lauric acid. It has a long shelf life. It has a "light" texture. Use for dryness, itching, sensitive skin, and as a tanning aid. Use as a base or 10-50% additive.
Adding Sweet Almond Oil increases both shelf life and wash ability.

**Evening Primrose Oil** - Use externally for psoriasis, eczema, and to aid in wound healing. Helps to prevent prematurely aged skin. Helps in healing scars. Contains gamma lineolenic acid, vitamins & minerals.

**Flax Seed Oil** - Use externally for oil skin and acne. Helps psoriasis, eczema, Helps to prevent scarring and stretch marks. Goes rancid quickly. Use as 10-50% additive. Contains EFA, GLA, Linolenic and oleic acid (Omega 3 and 9), vitamins and minerals.

**Grapeseed Oil -** Use for all skin types. Odorless, light, and penetrating. Slightly astringent, tightens and tones the skin. Does not aggravate acne. May use at full strength. Contains vitamins, minerals, protein, and linoleic acid.

**Hazelnut Oil -** Slightly astringent, toning, and fast absorbing. Use for oily skin, combination skins, and acne. Will tone and tighten skin and help maintain firmness and elasticity. May be useful against thread veins by tightening the capillaries Encourages cell regeneration & stimulates circulation Use 100% as base or in 10% dilution. Contains vitamins, minerals, proteins, oleic and linoleic acid.

**Jojoba Oil** - Not great for a massage oil, but very nourishing for the skin. It helps to heal inflamed skins, psoriasis, eczema, and dermatitis. Can help to control acnes and oily skin or scalp. Use for hair care. Good for all skin types but may clog pores. Can be used for arthritis/rheumatism Use at 10% dilution or full strength. This oil is a WAX. Contains protein, minerals, plant wax, and myristic acid (an anti-inflammatory).

**Olive Oil** - Use for rheumatic conditions, hair care, cosmetics, nails, acne, skin inflammations, bruises, and sprains. 10-50%.Contains protein, minerals, and vitamins. Very healing but has a strong odor.

**Peanut Oil** - BE VERY CAREFUL AS SOME PEOPLE ARE ALLERGIC. Good for all skin types, arthritis and sunburns. Good for massage. Contains protein, vitamins, minerals.

**Rose Hip Seed Oil** - Use for dry, scaly fissured skin, dull skin, acnes, eczema, psoriasis, burns, ulcerated veins and to fade old scars. DO NOT use on acne, blemished, or oily skin. Use neat or at 10% additive. Goes rancid very quickly. Contains GLA, Linolenic, Oleic, and Palmitic acids

**Safflower Oil** - Use for all skin types, sprains, bruises, inflamed joints.Light and Odorless. Turns rancid very quickly. Seldom used with oils. Contains proteins, vitamins, minerals, and linoleic acid.

**Sesame Oil** - Use for psoriasis, eczema, arthritis, rheumatism, tanning aid. A thick oil with strong odor. Use as base or 10% dilution. Contains vitamins, minerals, proteins, lecithin, amino acid.

**Wheat germ Oil** -Use for dry cracked skin, stretch marks, prematurely aged skin, eczema, psoriasis. Thick, sticky. Use 10% dilution. Contains proteins, minerals, vitamins E, A, and D. DO NOT use on those who have low blood pressure or low blood sugar levels. May cause skin irritation or elevate cholesterol levels in the body.

**Choosing your Essential Oil**

Listed on the next page is only a sampling of some of the more favorite essential oils that you can use to create the perfume blend of your dreams.

There are literally hundreds of essential oils available to the public. I have narrowed the search down to most affordable and widely used essential oils.

Be sure to jot down the essential oils that peak your interest and then compare them with the chart listing the Top, Middle and Bottom Notes. Then, make you choice from no more than 5 essential oils. Have fun and experiment.

When creating a perfume blend, always use a glass container. You can purchase fancy little bottles to put your blend in. At one time I collected several fancy bottles with fancy spray heads on them, just like the kind you would see in the old movies, at the dollar store. These made great gifts when I personalized them with one- of-a-kind perfume blends for the receiver.

Using glass also keeps the blend fresh. Keep your blends away from direct sunlight and heat sources. They will last longer this way.

**Short List of Essential Oils and their properties:**

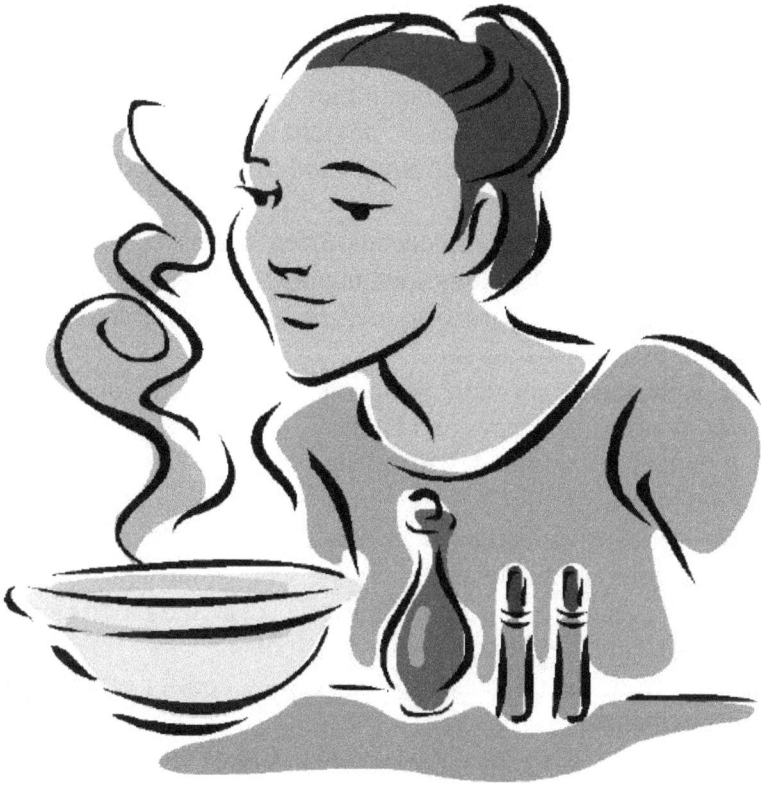

**Allspice**. Spicy top note warms the heart with memories of mama's kitchen.

**Amber/Ambergris**. Only used in synthetic form now as a fixative in perfumery. Oriental fragrance bringing out a warm and dramatic aroma.

**Angelica.** Musky odor often used as a fixative in perfumery. Aniseed-Relieves exhaustion, tension, depression and stress. Calms. Basil-Uplifting. Stimulates the adrenal cortex. Antidepressant. Bergamot-Relaxant or stimulant. Spicy citrus. Eases grieving.

**Cedarwood**-Calming. Avoid during pregnancy. Relieves tensions and stress. Woody fragrance.

**Chamomile**-Relieves and calms the mind. Brings mental clarity.

**Cinnamon**-A great stimulant and tonic. Do not use during pregnancy.

**Frankincense**-Sedative. Aids in meditation. Breaks cords that bind.

**Geranium**-Relieves tension and anxiety. Relaxant or stimulant. Antidepressant. Sweet and floral. Antidepressant. Relieves PMS.

**Jasmine**-Aphrodisiac and confidence booster. Makes a great erotic perfume blend. Develops and encourages creativity.

**Juniper**-Detoxifies and clears away negativity. Relieves anxiety, tension and stress. Spicy fragrance.

**Lavender**-Aphrodisiac for men. Relaxant or stimulant. Floral with woody notes. Balances and Harmonizes.

**Lemon**-Relaxant or stimulant. Citrus fragrance.

**Linden Blossom**-Light floral scent and is often used in perfume blends.

**Marjoram**-Relieves tension headaches and other tensions and stress. Eases grief and being alone. Warm, woody and spicy fragrance.

**Neroli**-Enhances the creative process. Erotic scent and mood elevator.

**Orange**-Uplifts and stimulates. Fresh citrus scent.

**Patchouli**-Aphrodisiac that has a strong scent. Good for centering and grounding.

**Peppermint**-Avoid using during pregnancy. Fights feelings of unworthiness and self doubt. Helps one to let go of ego.

**Petitgrain**-Sedative and antidepressant. Increases mental clarity. Woody and floral.

**Pine**-Relieves stress, tension, exhaustion and fatigue. Woody fragrance.

**Rose**-Aphrodisiac which helps to overcome frigidity and increases semen production. A real confidence builder and mood elevator. Brings thoughts of love.

**Rosemary**-Stimulating and energizing. Avoid using during pregnancy. Brings mental clarity.

**Sandalwood**-Relieves stress and tension. Calms the mind. Makes a great oriental or woody blend.

**Sage**-Sacred plant used in Native American smudging rituals. Brings strength and fortitude.

**Spearmint**-Refreshing and stimulating. Sweet smell.

**Spikenard**-Relaxant. Heavy and sweet woody and spicy odor. Blends well with spicy oils.

**Tuberose**-Aphrodisiac. Sweet and floral scent.

**Vanilla**-Calms and elevates the mood. A strong aphrodisiac. A very fragrant aroma.

**Vetiver**-Calms and cools the emotions. Centers and Grounds. Relieves depression and stress. Aroma of the earth.

**Ylang Ylang**-Relaxing and calming. Releases thoughts of anger and discord. Creates a space of peace and contentment. Considered an aphrodisiac. Sweet, light and floral scent.


**Contraindications**

- If you have seizures/epilepsy avoid the following oils:
    Fennel, Hyssop, Rosemary, Sage and Thyme.
- If you are Pregnant avoid the following oils:
    Aniseed, Angelic, Basil, Birch, Black Pepper, Camphor, Carrot Seed, Cassia, Cedarwood, Chamomile, Cinnamon, Clary Sage, Clove, Coriander, Fennel, Ginger, Hyssop, Jasmine, Juniper, Lemongrass, Marjoram, Melissa, Myrrh, Nutmeg, Oregano, Peppermint, Pine, Rockrose, Rose, Rosemary, Sage and Thyme.
- If you have High Blood Pressure avoid:
    Pine, Rosemary, Sage and Thyme.
- If you have Kidney Problems avoid:
    Juniper, Sandalwood and Coriander.
- Essential oils that can cause skin sensitivity or irritation:
    Allspice, Basil, Benzoin, Black Pepper, Cassia, Cinnamon Bark, Clove, Fennel, Ginger, Lemon, Lemongrass, Lemon Verbena, Oregano, Peppermint, Pine, Tagetes and Thym

**NOTES:**

**Chapter Fifteen**
**Making Floral Water**


**Making Floral Water**

Making floral water is both fun and inexpensive. You can use floral water in many ways including room sprays, aromatherapy blends, and even add to your bath water. Below is a simple recipe that I have used for years.


**Ingredients:**
    **2 cups of spring water**
    **1 cup of fresh flower blossoms**

1.  Find a large glass bowl and pour in the water.
2.  Bruise the flower blossoms. (You can accomplish this by placing the blossoms in a mortar bowl and using a pedestal to break the fibers of the blossoms.)
3.  Place a cheesecloth into the bowl of water and place the bruised flower blossoms on the cheesecloth being sure that the water covers the blossoms and that the edges of the cheesecloth are on the outside of the bowl.
4.  Cover the bowl and let it sit overnight-Or-set the bowl out in direct sunlight for 2-4 hours.
5.  When finished, pick up the edges of the cheesecloth and bring the edges together and lift the cheesecloth out of the water. Now gently squeeze the cheesecloth allowing the leftover water to drip back into the bowl.
6.  Take the bowl of water and pour it into a small pot and simmer it on the stove until there is only 1 teaspoon of the liquid left.
7.  Cool and place this teaspoon of liquid into a small glass bottle, preferably a dark or cobalt blue one.

Shelf life: 1 month

When making simple floral waters at home, there are two ways that you can choose to use.
1. Sun Method
2. Boiling Method

## 1.  Sun Method

Choose this method when the weather is nice and you have at least 2-4 hours of sunshine. The Sun Method works best for flower heads and blossoms while the Boiling Method works better for woodier plants. No matter which method you use, dilute the water with equal parts of brandy and pour into a glass bottle. This is the *mother tincture*. Label your mixture. To make a stock bottle, take two drops of the mother tincture and add it to 30ml of brandy.

What you will need:
Glass bowl
Spring or distilled water
Flowers

## To Do:

1. Wait for a sunny day and pour spring or distilled water into a glass bowl. Pick fresh flowers in full bloom (without any blemishes on them) and place them in the glass bowl of water.
2. I always ask permission to remove these blooms and to use them in making my remedies. It may sound to some as a silly thing to do, but I believe that we must always ask the plant permission to use them. It just feels like that right thing to do energetically speaking. Let the flowers float on top of the water covering the surface of the water in the bowl. Place the bowl in direct sunlight for 2-4 hours.
3. When sufficient time has passed, strain the flowers out of the water and pour the water into glass bottle along with ½ parts brandy (for preservation). This is your stock bottle. It may be difficult to find some of the Bach Flower plants where you live.

Below is an example of a flower that grows easily here in Florida, USA---

Impatiens.

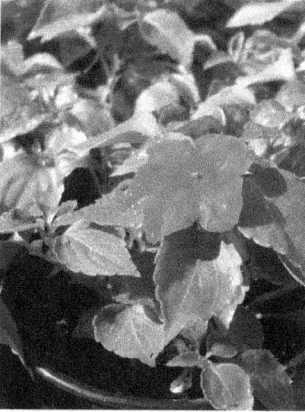

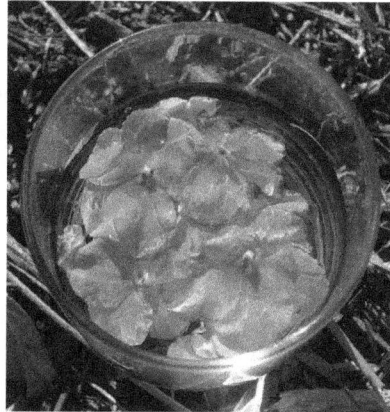

After picking the best flower tops from the plant, place in a glass container filled with spring water. You can make as much remedy as you want too. For illustration purposes, I used a small glass of water with a handful of flower petals as shown in the photo to the right.

After you have created your flower essence using the sun method, strain the flower material from the water and discard the petals. This jar is your flower essence. In another glass bottle, add equal part of flower essence to brandy (for preservation). Please be sure to label and date it.

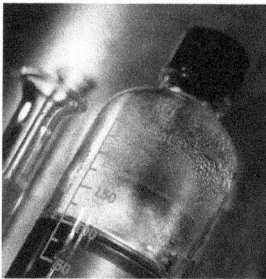

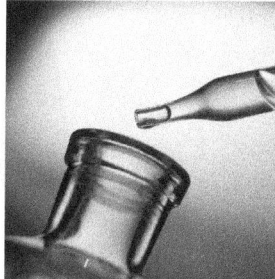

## 2. The Boiling Method

Use this method when the weather is not nice outside and you are not receiving at least 4 hours of sunlight. This method is also advisable to use for woodier plants. Also called the *'cooking method,'* this method requires that you place your flowers in a pot of water and place on the stove. Bring the water to a quick boil, turn off the heat and remove the pot from the hot burner. Allow the pot to cool down before you strain out the plant material and pour the water in a glass bottle. Add equal parts brandy to the bottle. This is your stock bottle.

What you will need:
Cooking Pot
Spring or distilled water
Flowers

## To Do:

Bring one cup of water to boil. Turn off heat and add one cup of flower petals to the cup of water. Let petals steep until water cools (15 minutes to 1 hour). Strain out petals and pour water (essence) into a glass container and label. Add equal parts of brandy and water (essence) to a glass bottle. This is your stock bottle.

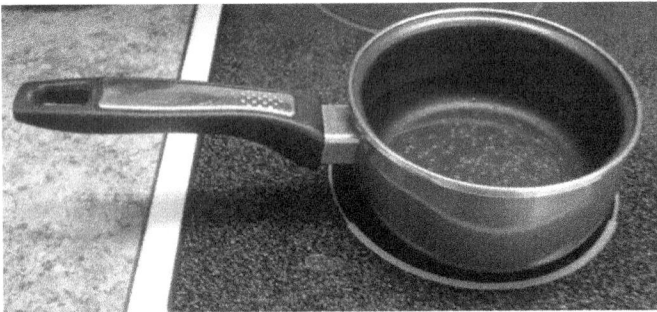

1. Bring water in pot to a full boil

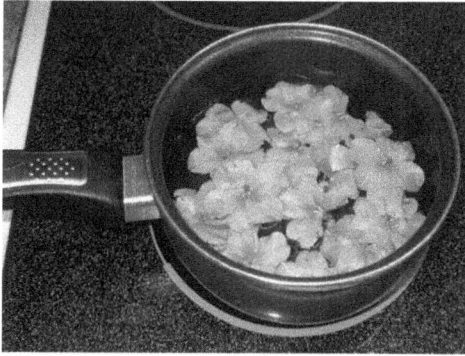

2. Toss in flower petals, turn off water and remove pot from burner. Let steep for 10-20 minutes. Allow mixture to cool before moving on to next level.

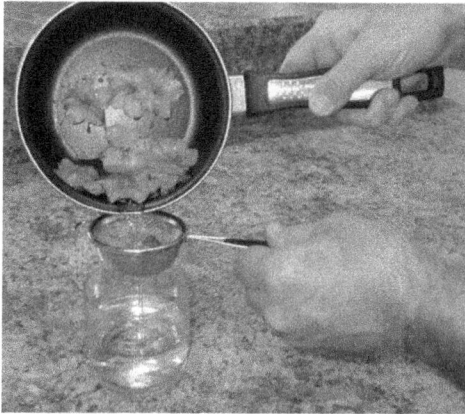

3. After mixture has cooled, strain petals from water into glass jar. Discard or compost petals. This jar is your flower essence.

　　In another glass bottle, add equal part of flower essence to brandy (for preservation). Please be sure to label and date it. This is your mother tincture.

**Great Flower Blossoms to Use to make Floral Water**

Frangipani
Gardenia
Geranium
Honeysuckle
Hyacinth
Lavender
Lilac
Magnolia
Marigold
Narcissus
Orange Blossoms
Honeysuckle Rose

**Chapter Sixteen**
**Some Recipes**

**How to make Perfumed Body Oil**

**#1 Coconut Body Oil Ingredients**:
> 4 teaspoons coconut oil
> 10-15 drops of essential oil
> 2 – 100 mg. of vitamin E capsules.

**To Do**:
Pour the coconut oil into a dark glass container and begin to add the essential oil drop by drop. Shake the blend after each drop and smell it. If you need more essential oils continue to place one drop of essential into the oil, shake it and smell it.

Continue this until you have found the perfect aroma.

Cut a slit into the two vitamin E capsules and squeeze the liquid into the blend. Discard the capsules. Shake well and smell again. If you are not pleased with the aroma, continue to add essential oils, shake and smell until you are.

Tighten cap on the container and place it in a cool dry place out of direct sunlight for 1-2 weeks.

**#2 Jojoba Body Oil Ingredients**:
    4 teaspoons Jojoba oil
    10-15 drops of essential oil

**To Do:**
Pour the jojoba oil into a dark glass container and begin to add the essential oil drop by drop. Shake the blend after each drop and smell it. If you need more essential oils continue to place one drop of essential into the oil, shake it and smell it.

Continue this until you have found the perfect aroma.

When you are pleased with the aroma of the body oil, then tighten the cap on the container and place it in a cool dry place out of direct sunlight for 1-2 weeks.

**Sample Perfume Formulas**

**Citrus Blend to uplift and energize Ingredients:**
>7 drops of Grapefruit 7 drops of Orange
>4 drops of Chamomile 3 drops of Neroli
>2 drops of narcissus 2 drops of vanilla
>2 drops of vanillin
>2 ounces of jojoba oil

**To Do:**
Pour the jojoba oil into a dark glass container and begin to add the essential oils drop by drop. Shake the blend after each drop and smell it. If you need more essential oils continue to place one drop of essential into the oil, shake it and smell it.

Continue this until you have found the perfect aroma.

When you are pleased with the aroma of the body oil, then tighten the cap on the container and place it in a cool dry place out of direct sunlight for 1-2 weeks.

Shelf Life: 6 months to 1 year

**Woody Blend for Seriousness Ingredients:**
>    7 drops of Petitgrain
>    4 drops of Rose Geranium 4 drops of Rosewood
>    drops of Coriander 4 drops of Melissa
>    drops of Juniper Berry 4 drops of Pine
>    2 drops of Cedarwood 1 ounces of Jojoba oil

**To Do:**
Pour the jojoba oil into a dark glass container and begin to add the essential oils drop by drop. Shake the blend after each drop and smell it. If you need more essential oils continue to place one drop of essential into the oil, shake it and smell it.

Continue this until you have found the perfect aroma.

When you are pleased with the aroma of the body oil, then tighten the cap on the container and place it in a cool dry place out of direct sunlight for 1-2 weeks.

Shelf Life: 6 months to 1 year

**Exotic and Memorable Nights Ingredients:**
　　7 drops of Sandalwood
　　7 drops Musk
　　6 drops of Frankincense
　　3 drops of Vanilla
　　2 drops of vanillin
　　2 teaspoons of jojoba oil

**To Do**:
Pour the jojoba oil into a dark glass container and begin to add the essential oils drop by drop. Shake the blend after each drop and smell it. If you need more essential oils continue to place one drop of essential into the oil, shake it and smell it.

Continue this until you have found the perfect aroma.

When you are pleased with the aroma of the body oil, then tighten the cap on the container and place it in a cool dry place out of direct sunlight for 1-2 weeks.

Shelf Life: 6 months to 1 year

**Remember Me Ingredients:**
 6 drops of Geranium
 4 drops of Lemongrass
 4 drops of Coriander
 3 drops of Rosewood
 3 drops of Patchouli
 3 drops of Palmarosa
 2 ounces of jojoba oil

**To Do:**
Pour the jojoba oil into a dark glass container and begin to add the essential oils drop by drop. Shake the blend after each drop and smell it. If you need more essential oils continue to place one drop of essential into the oil, shake it and smell it.

Continue this until you have found the perfect aroma.

When you are pleased with the aroma of the body oil, then tighten the cap on the container and place it in a cool dry place out of direct sunlight for 1-2 weeks.

Shelf Life: 6 months to 1 year

**Lingering Moments Ingredients:**
    9 drops of Marigold
    7 drops of Ginger
    7 drops of Rockrose
    2 drops of Lavender
    2 ounces of Jojoba Oil

**To Do:**
Pour the jojoba oil into a dark glass container and begin to add the essential oils drop by drop. Shake the blend after each drop and smell it. If you need more essential oils continue to place one drop of essential into the oil, shake it and smell it.

Continue this until you have found the perfect aroma.

When you are pleased with the aroma of the body oil, then tighten the cap on the container and place it in a cool dry place out of direct sunlight for 1-2 weeks.

Shelf Life: 6 months to 1 year

**Relax and Enjoy Ingredients:**
> drops of Carnation
> 6 drops of Tuberose
> 5 drops of Narcissus
> 3 drops of rose
> 3 drops of Ylang Ylang
> 3 drops of Lavender
> 2 ounces of jojoba oil

**To Do:**
Pour the jojoba oil into a dark glass container and begin to add the essential oils drop by drop. Shake the blend after each drop and smell it. If you need more essential oils continue to place one drop of essential into the oil, shake it and smell it.

Continue this until you have found the perfect aroma.

When you are pleased with the aroma of the body oil, then tighten the cap on the container and place it in a cool dry place out of direct sunlight for 1-2 weeks.

Shelf Life: 6 months to 1 year

**Oriental Nights Ingredients:**
>6 drops of Amber
>3 drops of Sandalwood
>3 drops of Frankincense
>3 drops of Resins
>3 drops of Musk
>3 drops of Ylang Ylang
> 3 drops of Lavender
>2 ounces of jojoba oil

**To Do:**
Pour the jojoba oil into a dark glass container and begin to add the essential oils drop by drop. Shake the blend after each drop and smell it. If you need more essential oils continue to place one drop of essential into the oil, shake it and smell it.

Continue this until you have found the perfect aroma.

When you are pleased with the aroma of the body oil, then tighten the cap on the container and place it in a cool dry place out of direct sunlight for 1-2 weeks.

Shelf Life: 6 months to 1 year

**Starry Night Unwinding Ingredients:**
    8 drops of Chamomile
    8 drops of Valerian
    4 drops Neroli
    3 drops of Lavender
    2 ounces of jojoba oil

**To Do**:
Pour the jojoba oil into a dark glass container and begin to add the essential oils drop by drop. Shake the blend after each drop and smell it. If you need more essential oils continue to place one drop of essential into the oil, shake it and smell it.

Continue this until you have found the perfect aroma.

When you are pleased with the aroma of the body oil, then tighten the cap on the container and place it in a cool dry place out of direct sunlight for 1-2 weeks.

Shelf Life: 6 months to 1 year

**Evoking Passion Ingredients:**
>6 drops of Passion Flower
>6 drops of Neroli
>4 drops of Narcissus
>3 drops of rose
>3 drops of Ylang Ylang
>3 drops of Lavender
>2 ounces of jojoba oil

**To Do:**
Pour the jojoba oil into a dark glass container and begin to add the essential oils drop by drop. Shake the blend after each drop and smell it. If you need more essential oils continue to place one drop of essential into the oil, shake it and smell it.

Continue this until you have found the perfect aroma.

When you are pleased with the aroma of the body oil, then tighten the cap on the container and place it in a cool dry place out of direct sunlight for 1-2 weeks.

Shelf Life: 6 months to 1 year

**Enchante' Ingredients:**
  10 drops of Sandalwood
  10 drops of Peony
  3 drops of Ylang Ylang
  3 drops of Lavender
  2 ounces of jojoba oil


**To Do:**
Pour the jojoba oil into a dark glass container and begin to add the essential oils drop by drop. Shake the blend after each drop and smell it. If you need more essential oils continue to place one drop of essential into the oil, shake it and smell it.

Continue this until you have found the perfect aroma.

When you are pleased with the aroma of the body oil, then tighten the cap on the container and place it in a cool dry place out of direct sunlight for 1-2 weeks.

Shelf Life: 6 months to 1 yea

**Chapter Seventeen**
**Perfume and the Zodiac**

**The Capricorn Blend Ingredients:**
> 6 drops of honeysuckle
> 4 drops of lilac
> 4 drops of tulip
> 2 drops of mimosa
> 1 drop of vetivert
> 2 drops of lavender
> 2 ounces of jojoba oil

**To Do:**

Pour the jojoba oil into a dark glass container and begin to add the essential oils drop by drop. Shake the blend after each drop and smell it. If you need more essential oils continue to place one drop of essential into the oil, shake it and smell it. Continue this until you have found the perfect aroma.

When you are pleased with the aroma of the body oil, then tighten the cap on the container and place it in a cool dry place out of direct sunlight for 1-2 weeks. Shelf Life: 6 months to 1 year.

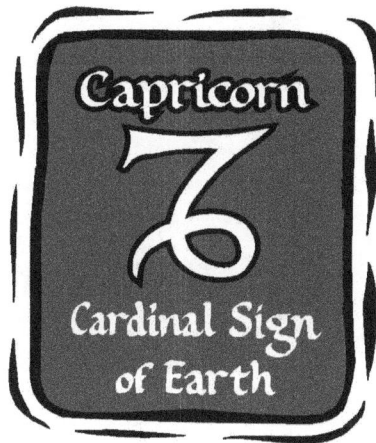

Capricorn
Cardinal Sign
of Earth

**The Aquarius Blend Ingredients:**
>7 drops of star anise
>7 drops of sweet pea
>2 drops of patchouli
>2 drops of ylang ylang
>2 drops of lavender
>2 ounces of jojoba oil

**To Do:**
Pour the jojoba oil into a dark glass container and begin to add the essential oils drop by drop. Shake the blend after each drop and smell it. If you need more essential oils continue to place one drop of essential into the oil, shake it and smell it. Continue this until you have found the perfect aroma.

When you are pleased with the aroma of the body oil, then tighten the cap on the container and place it in a cool dry place out of direct sunlight for 1-2 weeks. Shelf Life: 6 months to 1 year.

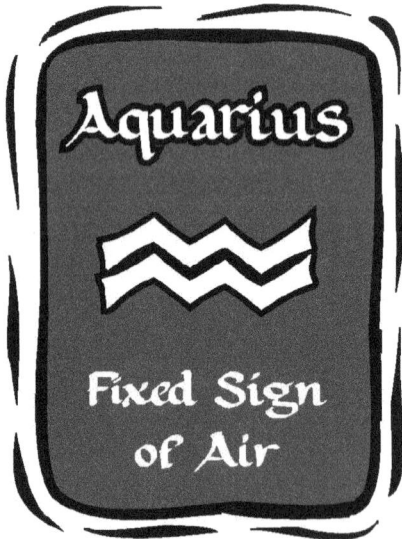

Aquarius

Fixed Sign
of Air

**The Pisces Blend Ingredients:**
8 drops of Jasmine
4 drops of Gardenia
4 drops of Hyacinth
2 drops of vanilla
2 drops of vanillin
2 drops of lavender
2 ounces of jojoba oil

**To Do:**
Pour the jojoba oil into a dark glass container and begin to add the essential oils drop by drop. Shake the blend after each drop and smell it. If you need more essential oils continue to place one drop of essential into the oil, shake it and smell it. Continue this until you have found the perfect aroma.

When you are pleased with the aroma of the body oil, then tighten the cap on the container and place it in a cool dry place out of direct sunlight for 1-2 weeks. Shelf Life: 6 months to 1 year.

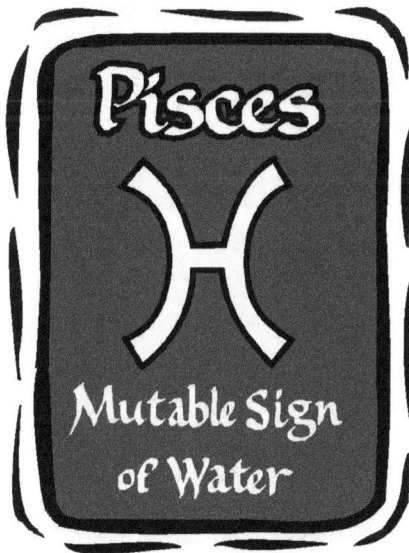

**The Aries Blend Ingredients:**

    8 drops of ginger
    8 drops of neroli
    3 drops of petitgrain
    3 drops of coriander
    1 drops of pine
    1 drop of black pepper
    2 drops of ylang ylang
    2 ounces of jojoba oil

**To Do:**

Pour the jojoba oil into a dark glass container and begin to add the essential oils drop by drop. Shake the blend after each drop and smell it. If you need more essential oils continue to place one drop of essential into the oil, shake it and smell it. Continue this until you have found the perfect aroma.

When you are pleased with the aroma of the body oil, then tighten the cap on the container and place it in a cool dry place out of direct sunlight for 1-2 weeks. Shelf Life: 6 months to 1 year.

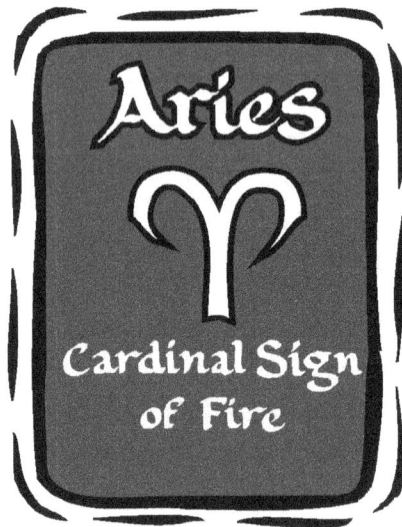

**The Taurus Blend Ingredients:**
> 6 drops of magnolia
> 6 drops of honeysuckle
> 4 drops of lilac
> 2 drops of plumeria
> 2 drops of rose
> 2 drops of ylang ylang
> 2 ounces of jojoba oil

**To Do:**

Pour the jojoba oil into a dark glass container and begin to add the essential oils drop by drop. Shake the blend after each drop and smell it. If you need more essential oils continue to place one drop of essential into the oil, shake it and smell it. Continue this until you have found the perfect aroma.

When you are pleased with the aroma of the body oil, then tighten the cap on the container and place it in a cool dry place out of direct sunlight for 1-2 weeks. Shelf Life: 6 months to 1 year.

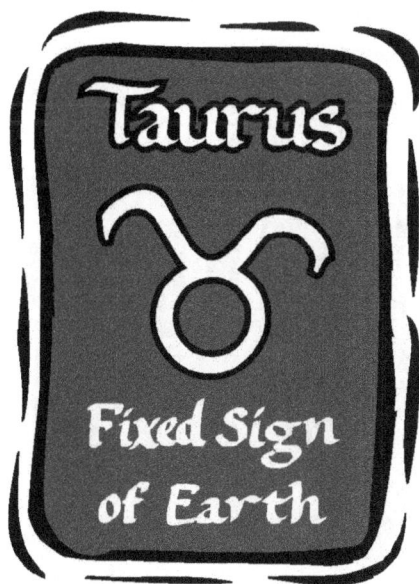

**The Gemini Blend Ingredients:**

      7 drops of bergamot
      1 drops of peppermint
      3 drops of dill
      3 drops of caraway
      3 drops of sweet pea
      3 drops of lemongrass
      3 drops of lily of the valley
      3 drops of lavender
      2 ounces of jojoba oil

**To Do:**

Pour the jojoba oil into a dark glass container and begin to add the essential oils drop by drop. Shake the blend after each drop and smell it. If you need more essential oils continue to place one drop of essential into the oil, shake it and smell it. Continue this until you have found the perfect aroma.

When you are pleased with the aroma of the body oil, then tighten the cap on the container and place it in a cool dry place out of direct sunlight for 1-2 weeks. Shelf Life: 6 months to 1 year.

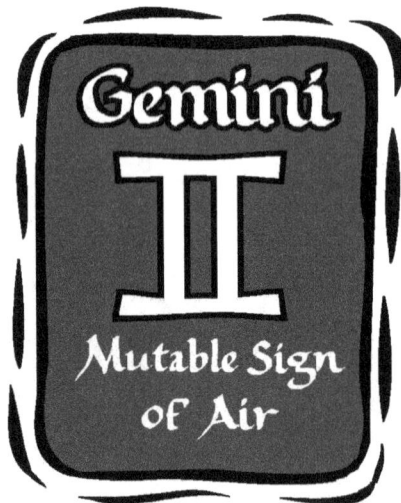

Gemini

Mutable Sign of Air

**The Cancer Blend Ingredients**:
- 10 drops of jasmine
- 4 drops of rose
- 3 drops of plumeria
- 3 drops of palmarosa
- 2 drops of chamomile
- 3 drops of ylang ylang
- 2 ounces of jojoba oil

**To Do:**

Pour the jojoba oil into a dark glass container and begin to add the essential oils drop by drop. Shake the blend after each drop and smell it. If you need more essential oils continue to place one drop of essential into the oil, shake it and smell it.     Continue this until you have found the perfect aroma.

When you are pleased with the aroma of the body oil, then tighten the cap on the container and place it in a cool dry place out of direct sunlight for 1-2 weeks. Shelf Life: 6 months to 1 year.

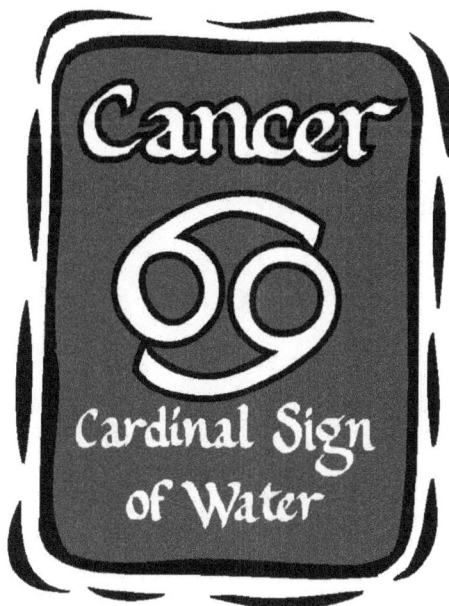

Cancer
Cardinal Sign of Water

## The Leo Blend Ingredients:

 7 drops of cinnamon
 5 drops of ginger
 4 drops of nasturtium
 3 drops of neroli
 2 drops of orange
 1 drops of petitgrain
 1 drops of frankincense
 2 drops of ylang ylang
 2 ounces of jojoba oil

## To Do:

Pour the jojoba oil into a dark glass container and begin to add the essential oils drop by drop. Shake the blend after each drop and smell it. If you need more essential oils continue to place one drop of essential into the oil, shake it and smell it. Continue this until you have found the perfect aroma.

When you are pleased with the aroma of the body oil, then tighten the cap on the container and place it in a cool dry place out of direct sunlight for 1-2 weeks. Shelf Life: 6 months to 1 year.

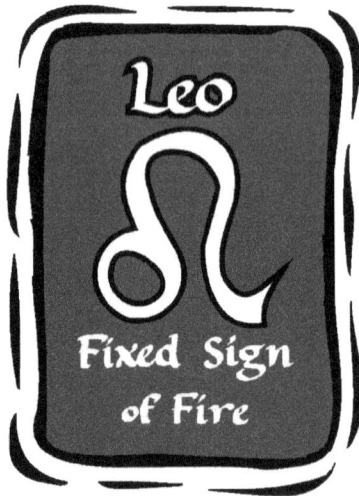

**The Virgo Blend Ingredient**:
      8 drops of honeysuckle
      3 drops of fennel
      3 drops of oak moss
      3 drops of patchouli
      3 drops of clary sage
      2 drops of caraway
      1 drop of fennel
      2 drops of lavender
      2 ounces of jojoba oil

**To Do:**

Pour the jojoba oil into a dark glass container and begin to add the essential oils drop by drop. Shake the blend after each drop and smell it. If you need more essential oils continue to place one drop of essential into the oil, shake it and smell it. Continue this until you have found the perfect aroma.

When you are pleased with the aroma of the body oil, then tighten the cap on the container and place it in a cool dry place out of direct sunlight for 1-2 weeks. Shelf Life: 6 months to 1 year.

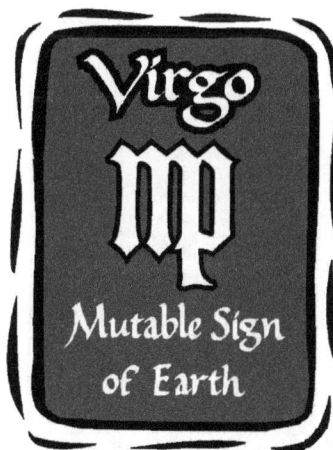

Virgo

♍

Mutable Sign
of Earth

**The Libra Blend Ingredient**:

      3 drops of roman chamomile
      3 drops of daffodil
      3 drops of dill
      3 drops of palmarosa
      2 drops of fennel
      1 drop of geranium
      1 drop of peppermint
      2 drops of vanilla
      2 ounces of jojoba oil

**To Do:**

Pour the jojoba oil into a dark glass container and begin to add the essential oils drop by drop. Shake the blend after each drop and smell it. If you need more essential oils continue to place one drop of essential into the oil, shake it and smell it. Continue this until you have found the perfect aroma.

When you are pleased with the aroma of the body oil, then tighten the cap on the container and place it in a cool dry place out of direct sunlight for 1-2 weeks. Shelf Life: 6 months to 1 year.

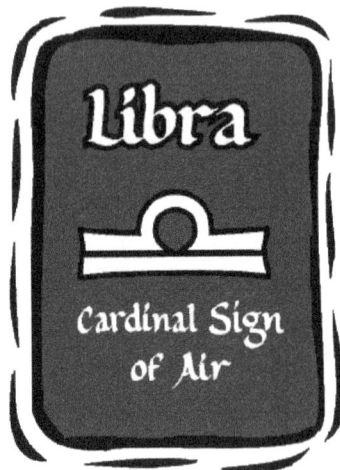

Libra

Cardinal Sign
of Air

**The Scorpio Blend Ingredient**:

    3 drops of black pepper
    3 drops of hyacinth
    3 drops of tuberose
    3 drops of pennyroyal
    2 drops of cardamon
    1 drop of thyme
    1 drop of pine
    2 ounces of jojoba oil

**To Do:**

Pour the jojoba oil into a dark glass container and begin to add the essential oils drop by drop. Shake the blend after each drop and smell it. If you need more essential oils continue to place one drop of essential into the oil, shake it and smell it. Continue this until you have found the perfect aroma.

When you are pleased with the aroma of the body oil, then tighten the cap on the container and place it in a cool dry place out of direct sunlight for 1-2 weeks. Shelf Life: 6 months to 1 year.

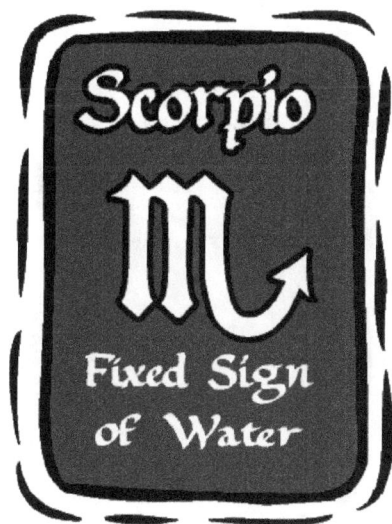

Scorpio
Fixed Sign
of Water

**The Sagittarius Blend Ingredient**:

   3 drops of bergamot
   3 drops of calendula
   3 drops of clove
   3 drops of lemon balm
   1 drops of nutmeg
   1 drop of oak moss
   1 drop of rosemary
   1 drop of saffron
   2 ounces of jojoba oil

**To Do:**

   Pour the jojoba oil into a dark glass container and begin to add the essential oils drop by drop. Shake the blend after each drop and smell it. If you need more essential oils continue to place one drop of essential into the oil, shake it and smell it. Continue this until you have found the perfect aroma.

   When you are pleased with the aroma of the body oil, then tighten the  cap on the container and place it in a cool dry place out of direct sunlight for 1-2 weeks. Shelf Life: 6 months to 1 year

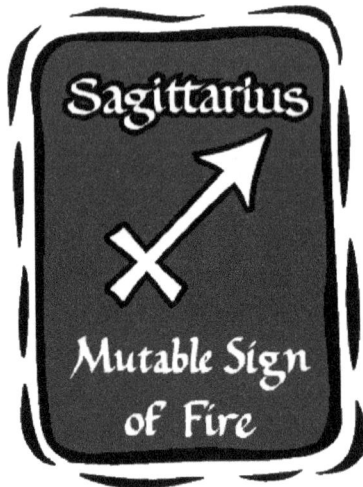

## Other Ways to Use your Blend

- Spray a little of your blend on a cotton ball or sheet of paper and place the ball, or paper, in your dresser drawers.
- Spray a little of your blend in your automobile for a more enjoyable trip.
- Spray a little of your blend on stationary or note cards.
- Spray a little of the blend on the gift wrapping paper, ribbon, or even the tag.
- Spray a little of the blend on a tissue and place in your purse, handbag, or suitcase.
- Spray a little of your blend on a cool light bulb. When you turn the light on, the heat from the bulb will slowly begin to release the scent.
- Spray a little of the blend on a candle. As the candle burns it will release the scent.
- Spray a little of the blend in your garbage cans and waste baskets to keep them smelling fresh.
- Spray a little of the blend on a softener sheet that you can toss into the dryer to give your clothes a wonderful scent.
- Spray a little of the blend on your guest towels, robes or slippers.
- Spray a little of the blend on your wrap, sweater or coat. Then when you need a little extra warmth and comfort around you, it will be there.
- Spray a little of the blend on a piece of cloth and tuck it into your pocket. Whenever you are feeling stressed, just pull out the cloth and take a whiff.
- Planning a romantic evening? Then please do spray the couch and/or bedroom pillows lightly with your favorite blend for a memorable experience.

## Glossary of Terms

Analgesic: Pain relieving. Agent or remedy that helps to deaden pain.
Antibacterial: Destroys bacteria
Antifungal: Destroys fungus and mold
Anti-inflammatory (Antiphlogistic): Reduces inflammation
Antispasmodic: Relieves spasms and cramping
Antiviral: Destroys viruses
Aphrodisiac: Promotes sexual desire
Carminative: Expulsion of gas from the intestines
Cholagogue: Elimination of bile from the gall bladder, bile ducts
Cicatrizant:  Promotes healing by scar formation at the location of a healing wound
Decongestant: Expels excess fluid in sinuses, tissues and membranes
Deodorant: Eliminates body odors
Diaphoretic: Increases perspiration or sweat
Emmenahogue: Promotes menstruation
Expectorant: Promotes expulsion of mucus
Febrifuge: Fever reducing
Hepatic: Relating to the liver. Relaxes the liver and tones and aids its function.
Nervine: Supports and strengthens the nervous system and nerves
Purgative: Stimulates the movement of the bowels
Relaxant: Calms or relaxes nerves, organ, body and/or mind
Rubefacient: Causes redness of the skin
Stimulant: Increases circulation, movements of body, mind or spirit
Stomachic: Stomach stimulant or tonic, improves appetite
Vulnerary: Heals Wounds and sores by external application

## About the Author

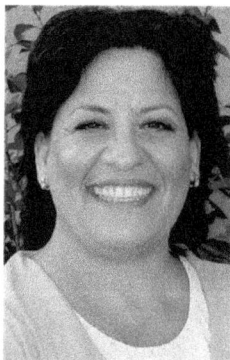

**Francine Milford, BS, LMT, CTN**

Francine Milford, BS, LMT, CTN, is a state and nationally licensed massage therapist and personal trainer who resides in Venice, Florida where she is the owner of the Reiki Center of Venice. At the Center, Francine teaches more than 70 different modalities of Alternative Therapies which include Bach Flower, Aromatherapy, Herbology, Homeopathy, Chakra Energy Work and Reiki Natural System of Healing.

Francine is a continuing education provider for the National Certifying Board of Therapeutic Massage and Bodywork (NCBTMB) and BOC, the National Athletic Trainers Association, as well as, for the State of Florida Massage Therapy Board.

The Reiki Center of Venice offers two levels of Aromatherapy Correspondence Courses a total 250 hour program of professional study. Level One is 50 hours in length and Level Two is 200 hours of training.

To learn more about this wonderful course which is easy to understand and with directions that is easy to follow, order yours today. You can view what is included in your purchase on the website before you make your decision. This course is the best priced course on the market today. You won't be sorry you did. Visit www.AromaCareBooks.com.

## References

Badcock, Laura (2008, Dec. 18). *Absorption & elimination of essential oils.* Web. Retrieved from http://www.essentialwholesale.com/library/absorption-elimination-of-essential-oils.

Battaglia, S. (2003). *The complete guide to aromatherapy.* 2nd ed. The Perfect Potion. Pty Ltd.

Buckle, J. (2003). *Clinical aromatherapy: Essential oils in practice, 2nd Ed.* Edinburgh: Churchill Livingstone.

Cooksley, Valerie Gennari. (1996). *Aromatherapy: a lifetime guide to healing with essential oils.* Prentice Hall.

Halcón, Linda and Maher, Kater. (2013, July 16). *How do I determine the quality of essential oils.* The University of Minnesota. Web. Retrieved from http://www.takingcharge.csh.umn.edu/explore-healing-practices/aromatherapy/how-do-i-determine-quality-essential-oils.

Hochell, Jennifer. (2006). *Introduction to Aromatherapy.* Home Study Course and Certification.

Hochell, Jennifer. (2006). *Advanced Aromatherapy.* Home Study Course and Certification.

Jones L. (1998) "Establishing standards for essential oils and analytical standards" *Proceedings of NAHA The World of Aromatherapy II International Conference and Trade Show* St. Louis, Missouri, Sept 25-28, 1998, p146-163.

Lawless, Julia. (1997). *The complete illustrated guide to aromatherapy, a practical approach to the use of essential oils for health and well-being.* Element Books Limited.

Lawless, Julia. (1995). *The illustrated encyclopedia of essential oils, the complete guide to the use of oils in aromatherapy and herbalism.* Element Books Limited.

Lyth, Geoff. 2002. *Sources and origins of our essential oils.* Quinessence Aromatherapy. Retrieved from http://www.quinessence.com/essential_oil_origins.htm.

Margaret, Ingrid. (2006). *Aromatherapy for massage practitioners.* Lippincott Williams & Wilkins.

Price, S. & Price, L. (2007). Aromatherapy for health professionals, 3rd
    Ed. Philadelphia: Churchill Livingstone Elsevier.
    Salvo, Susan. (2007). *Massage therapy principles and practice.*
    3rd Edition. Saunders Elsevier.
Salvo, Susan. (2007). *Massage therapy principles and practice.* 3rd
    Edition. Saunders Elsevier.
Shannon, J.C. (2012, August 7). *Curbing cravings and assaulting
    addictions with essential oils.* Web. Retrieved from
    http://essentialhealth.com/2012/08/curbing-cravings-and-
    assaulting-addictions-with-essential-oils.
Thibodeau and Patton. (2008). *Structure and function of the body.* 13th
    ed. Mosby, Inc.
    Tisserand, R. & Balacs, T. (1995). *Essential oil safety: A guide for
    health professionals.* Edinburgh: Churchill Livingstone.
U.S. Food and Drug Administration (FDA). (2009). Fragrances in
    Cosmetics. Web. Retrieved from
    http://www.fda.gov/Cosmetics/ProductsIngredients.
Williams, D.G. (1997). *The chemistry of essential oils: an introduction
    for aromatherapists, beauticians, retailers and students.* England:
    Micelle Press.
Worwood, Valerie Ann. (1991). *The complete book of essential oils &
    aromatherapy.* New World Library.

**Websites:**
Visit www.AromaCareBooks.com for sfree information, tips and blends.
Visit www.ReikiCenterofVenice.com for upcoming classes and health
articles.
Visit www.Naha.org for information on Aromatherapy